Dr. Neumann's Guide to the

New Sexually Transmitted Diseases

Dr. Neumann's Guide to the

New Sexually Transmitted Diseases

Hans H. Neumann, M.D.
and Sylvia Simmons

ACROPOLIS BOOKS LTD.
WASHINGTON, D.C.

ACROPOLIS BOOKS, LTD.
Colortone Building, 2400 17th St., N.W.,
Washington, D.C. 20009

Printed in the United States of America by
COLORTONE PRESS
Creative Graphics, Inc.
Washington, D.C. 20009

Attention: Schools and Corporations
ACROPOLIS books are available at quantity discounts with bulk purchase for educational, business, or sales promotional use. For information, please write to: SPECIAL SALES DEPARTMENT, ACROPOLIS BOOKS LTD., 2400 17th ST., N.W., WASHINGTON, D.C. 20009.

Are there Acropolis Books you want but cannot find in your local stores?
You can get any Acropolis book title in print. Simply send title and retail price, plus $2.00 per copy to cover mailing and handling costs for each book desired. District of Columbia residents add applicable sales tax. Enclose check or money order only, no cash please, to: ACROPOLIS BOOKS LTD., 2400 17th ST., N.W., WASHINGTON, D.C. 20009.

Library of Congress Cataloging in Publication Data
Neumann, Hans H.
  Dr. Neumann's Guide to the new sexually transmitted diseases.
  Includes index.
  1. Sexually transmitted diseases—Popular works.
I. Simmons, S. H. (Sylvia H.) II. Title.
III. Title: Guide to the new sexually transmitted diseases.
[DNLM: 1. Venereology—Popular works. WC 140 N492d]
RC200.2.N47   1987   616.95'1   87-18682
ISBN 0-87491-874-X (pbk.)

Table of Contents

Introduction

For sixteen years, in my capacity as director of preventive medicine for the health departments of various urban/suburban areas in Connecticut, I have been involved in the diagnosis, treatment, and prevention of sexually transmitted diseases for a heterogeneous population that includes people of all ages, all races, both sexes, the gay community, and all income levels.

The clinics I directed were visited by some ten thousand patients a year. Obviously, I didn't speak to all of them personally, but various members of our staff did. I did have contact with a great number of these patients and with thousands more in earlier years when the S.T.D. epidemic began to mushroom throughout the country. In addition, during my years as a private practitioner, I treated so many cases of these diseases that I long ago lost count. As a lecturer at colleges, high schools, and various community groups, I had frequent occasion to speak with still others who have some personal interest in these diseases.

When I talk to people who have a sexually transmitted disease, or to sexually active adults who have no S.T.D. but are interested in the subject, or are frightened by the possibility of acquiring one, I never cease to be amazed at the lack of information, as well as the misinformation they have managed to pick up. Since we have learned a great deal in recent years about diagnosing, assessing, and successfully treating many of the venereal diseases, it seemed to me that it might be helpful to put into an easy-to-read book the answers to those questions about S.T.D.s that come up most frequently.

Whenever I could do so, I have tried to make the information less technical in order to make it readily understandable. If the material in some chapters appears to be more elementary than in others, it is because this book is directed to people of all ages with all levels of knowledge on this subject. At the end of the book, I have included a glossary of medical terms having to do with S.T.D.s.

I've not tried to make this a medical book, nor is it a textbook. However, there is adequate information in these pages for anyone interested in the basic facts about S.T.D.s: what they are, how you get them, how to prevent them, and how, to the extent currently possible, to get rid of them. I have not tried to sugarcoat the facts; nor, on the other hand, have I tried to scare anyone. If you're old enough to know about sex, you're old enough to have the straight story.

Much has changed in the last few years, since the eruption of the AIDS epidemic. Though frightening, it should not preoccupy one to the point of losing respect for other epidemic and treatable S.T.D.s. Without being as threatening as AIDS, they can, if ignored, cause a great deal of lasting damage.

Here, then, is the straight story on sexually transmitted diseases.

Hans H. Neumann, M.D.

CHAPTER ONE

S.T.D. Primer

What Everyone Should Know

Throughout this book you will be seeing the initials S.T.D., or S.T.D.s, which stand for sexually transmitted disease or diseases. Of course you know that V.D. stands for venereal disease. Both refer to infectious diseases that, ordinarily, spread from one person to another through sexual intercourse, or other intimate body contact. But, while V.D. traditionally encompasses only gonorrhea, syphilis, and three more rare diseases mentioned on the next page, S.T.D.s cover a broader spectrum. Obviously, there's some overlapping in these terms—the S.T.D.s *include* gonorrhea and syphilis. But the reverse is not true: when we speak of the S.T.D.s we also include a number of common ailments which are not, medically speaking, venereal diseases. More about this later on.

The "New" Sexually Transmitted Diseases

In recent years, there have been virtual epidemics of diseases transmitted through sexual contact, such as those caused by the herpes virus, the AIDS virus, chlamydia trachomatis, a type of mycoplasma, cytomegalovirus, and others. As infections, they are, except for AIDS, as old as syphilis and gonorrhea. But their incidence, and our knowledge of how widely prevalent they are, has greatly increased. Gonorrhea and syphilis have old familiar faces. These other infections are more difficult to diagnose and treat, giving them every opportunity to flourish and spread. Both medically and in common parlance, these diseases are referred to as the "new" S.T.D.s, not because they have just been discovered, but because they have only recently achieved epidemic proportions.

As I said, when in the past we spoke of venereal disease, we almost always meant gonorrhea or syphilis. Three other infections, rarely seen by physicians, have usually been included in the term V.D. They are chancroid, granuloma inguinale, and lymphogranulum venereum, but it's unlikely that you'll ever have to know or pronounce those names.

Of course, any communicable disease can be transmitted through the closeness of sexual contact. Even the flu or streptococcal sore throat can be passed along through such activity. However, the term S.T.D. usually refers to a more limited number of infections, those that are often, but not necessarily, associated with sexual intercourse. Included would be some types of herpes and chlamydial infections, discussed in Chapters 2 and 4.

From Venus, Venereal

The word "venereal" is a downer. Too bad—it shouldn't be. The word originally came from Venus, the goddess of love. Logically, then, having a venereal illness should mean "lovesick." Unfortunately, it doesn't. Of course, it's possible to be lovesick and have a venereal disease at the same time—but the combination doesn't make for much happiness.

The Most Common S.T.D.

Currently, the most widely found sexually transmitted organism is called chlamydia (the full, scientific name is chlamydia trachomatis). Chapter 4 describes the symptoms and treatment for this disease. This may come as a surprise to you, but chlamydia is more common than gonorrhea. We don't have exact statistics on how many cases occur each year, but it's apparent to the medical community that it now holds the number one spot in terms of prevalence.

You might be interested in knowing why we don't have more exact figures on chlamydia, as we do on gonorrhea and syphilis. The latter two are what we call "reportable" diseases—clinics and private physicians must file reports with their state health departments on how many cases they see. Since a chlamydia infection is not a reportable disease, we draw our statistical conclusions from shared reports within the medical community, taken from local and area-wide surveys. These reports tell us that the incidence of chlamydia varies a great deal among the different social strata. For example, it is relatively common in college populations.

Chlamydia is one of the organisms that in men causes non-gonococcal urethritis, an ailment with gonorrhea-like symptoms, including frequent urination, a discharge, and either burning or itching. In women, it may produce no symptoms at all that they might be aware of, even though it can cause an inflammation of the cervix—the tip of the womb. It can also cause an inflammation of the tubes and a number of other problems elsewhere in the body. I'll talk more about this later on in the chapter on chlamydial infections.

While chlamydial infections are the most common S.T.D.s of consequence, syphilis is—after AIDS—the most serious of them. By "serious" I mean that this infection, if untreated, can have devastating effects on the body and mind. Other infections, however, including gonorrhea, can also become serious and, on rare occasions, deadly.

It is possible for someone to have two, or even more, of the S.T.D.s at the same time. In fact, this happens rather often. Gonococcal and chlamydial infections are frequently acquired on the same occasion. Early syphilis and herpes can also appear together, confusing the picture and making a quick, visual diagnosis risky. These are just two examples of the many combinations I see in my clinics.

While chlamydial infections are perhaps the most prevalent among S.T.D.s, gonorrhea is the most common of the *reportable* diseases. The prevalence of herpes is also exceedingly high. Another surprise to most laypersons is the fact that syphilis is not as uncommon as it should be, considering the effective treatment methods available. Today we have more syphilis in the U.S. than measles or tuberculosis. This is a recent development.

Increasing Prevalence of S.T.D.s

There are several reasons why S.T.D.s are more prevalent nowadays than in the early sixties and fifties. Some of these reasons are sociological, related to contemporary patterns of behavior and life styles. Others, oddly enough, have been linked to medical progress.

Both physically and emotionally, young people mature earlier than they did in previous generations—much of this early behavioral maturing is due to television, the movies, and more sophisticated education. Given this early coming of age, along with a decrease in inhibitions since the end of World War II, people in this country and in many other western societies are starting their sexual activities earlier.

To some extent, the increased use of alcohol, marijuana, and hard drugs has contributed to the decrease in inhibitions about sex; inhibitions that have, in other times, been strong. At the same time, the average age of marriage has gone up, leaving the unmarried free for longer periods of time to experiment with new partners.

Because our mores regarding sex have changed, and with the number of divorces skyrocketing, sexually active people in our culture change partners more frequently than they did in other eras. It follows, therefore, that those who have S.T.D.s give them to a wider circle of people.

Unwittingly, medical progress was a major factor in the increase in S.T.D.s; advances in contraception allowed for a greater degree of preparedness and served to increase sexual activity, especially among young women. With fear of pregnancy no longer a strong deterrent to sex, and with the prevailing acceptance of experimentation with different partners, the likelihood of acquiring an infection increased greatly. However, the recent emergence of AIDS has altered this aspect of the sexual revolution and many sexually active people are now seeking monogamous relationships.

Through the years, fear of infection has always acted as a deterrent to promiscuity. Many a person shied away from casual sexual encounters for fear of V.D. Then we went through a period when it was thought that penicillin was a magic potion that could make an S.T.D. more quickly curable than a case of athlete's foot. This, in turn, led to a loss of respect for these infections and contributed to the sort of casual relationships that increase the possibility of infection.

Today, the fear of infection has, to a degree, returned—but not as much as one might expect. We know this from statistics that show only a moderate decline in the incidence of syphilis and gonorrhea.

S.T.D. At Epidemic Proportions

S.T.D.s have reached epidemic proportions the world over—with the notable exception of China—and the problem is grave enough to cause serious concern.

By no means are all AIDS, gonorrhea, and syphilis cases actually reported; far more cases occur than are indicated by official statistics. Reporting procedures throughout the world range from excellent to nonexistent, depending on the country.

In recent years, the rates of infection per thousand people in the U.S. decreased slightly for gonorrhea. Still, almost 900,000 cases are reported annually, although there are probably two to three times that number. Thirty thousand syphilis cases per year are reported. The number of other infections seems unchanged, except for AIDS.

The Centers for Disease Control (CDC), the national government agency which tracks epidemics, believes that there are many millions of people in this country suffering from genital herpes. One of the problems in tracking and treating S.T.D.s is that there may be additional millions of people who comprise a "silent reservoir"—they are carriers of the various infectious agents who are unaware of their infections. These people are spreading the diseases as fast as new sexual contacts are made.

The large number of cases and the once rare but now common complications have become a matter of public attention and concern. Aside from AIDS, there is particular concern about the possibility of inflammation of the tubes in women and the sperm ducts in men, either of which can produce sterility.

Other complications include a certain type of arthritis, endocarditis (an inflammation of the inner lining of the heart), and infections of the conjunctivae, which can affect the eyeball and vision. These are but a few of the many possible complications that can arise from untreated S.T.D.s, and when you add them to the fact that a newborn infant may be infected at birth, you can see that the problem, on a national and global scale, is a major one.

Risk Factors In S.T.D.s

Anyone who has sexual contact with a person infected with a communicable disease can get it. There are no limitations of age, color, sex, or social level, even though the opportunities may differ, group to group. Unless you're living in a one-to-one relationship with someone who is similarly monogamous, you are a potential target for an S.T.D. There is no such thing as natural immunity to such communicable diseases—if you're a member of the human race, that's good enough for these organisms. Some people become infected more readily and more violently than do others, with the symptoms and severity varying from person to person, depending on individual susceptibility factors. But anyone can get such an infection, given the opportunity.

However, in medicine we speak of "increased risk factors." For example, in coronary disease, such increased risk factors would be high blood pressure, smoking, high salt intake, obesity, etc. In S.T.D.s we can list six such factors:

(1) Youth. The highest prevalence of S.T.D.s occurs in people between eighteen and thirty years of age. Obviously, it does not begin suddenly at eighteen and end abruptly at thirty. A statistical curve showing the incidence of infections would decline gradually before eighteen and after thirty.

(2) Use of alcohol and drugs, including soft drugs. Because inhibitions recede when one is high, there is less caution exercised about the choice of sex partners.

(3) Low socio-economic level. Some people question whether this factor isn't really a statistical distortion because clinics are more likely to report V.D. than are private physicians. However, examinations and large-scale screening programs among private practitioners, as well as in clinics, have supported this as a risk factor.

(4) Male homosexuality. In the past, this segment of the population showed a greater willingness to take risks, including the risk of contracting an S.T.D. through intercourse with a partner of short acquaintance, whose sex habits and medical history were unknown. Furthermore, allowing for many individual exceptions, the rate of turnover in sexual partners was, and to some degree still is, generally greater among male homosexuals than among heterosexuals.

(5) Tattoos. This is a strange risk factor, and the reasons are open to speculation, but it's a fact that tattooed persons are more likely to have S.T.D.s than non-tattooed persons.

(6) Travel. In my clinical experience, and that of others who have reported on this risk factor, two-thirds of those in the middle-aged, middle-class range who have S.T.D.s acquired the infections while traveling—while at conventions, or on other away-from-home business trips. This is so common, in fact, that in our clinic, we speak of *conventional* gonorrhea.

Looking for Clues Before Intimacy

Unfortunately, there are no revealing clues by which you can make a snap diagnosis on whether a person with whom you're about to be intimate has an S.T.D. Even an expert can be fooled by superficial signs, unless he does a smear test (a small amount of discharge put on a slide, dried, stained, and examined under a microscope), a culture (the specimen is put on a medium which supports the growth of bacteria, if present, in the atmosphere of an incubator), a blood test, and other examinations. It's both unfair and unsafe for the non-trained person to jump to conclusions. For example, a skin rash, which could suggest syphilis or AIDS, might be a perfectly harmless condition. On the other hand, at various stages of the disease, neither one shows any outward signs at all.

In fact, many women and some men infected with an S.T.D. are unaware of it until some complication sets in, or until it is brought to their attention by a sex partner or a doctor. A man is more likely to know if he carries certain infections (frequency and pain of urination often alert the male sufferer), but even men can't be sure without testing, or what we call *screening* for S.T.D.s.

How One Acquires An S.T.D.—Debunking Some Myths

Sophisticated as people today may seem about the subject of sex, some old myths about the ways these diseases can be transmitted still persist. There are people who still believe that venereal diseases can be transmitted without sexual contact— for instance, from sitting in unclean bathtubs, touching dirty doorknobs, or from using contaminated eating utensils. Not so. In theory this is possible, but not practically speaking. The organisms causing these diseases are quite fragile and don't survive readily outside the body. Heat, cold, and drying up all discourage survival.

Physicians get some odd stories from patients who want to cover up, sometimes unconsciously, the source of their infection. Most doctors are discreet enough not to challenge such tales. But the truth of the matter is that the doorknob and the toilet seat are innocent. Workers in S.T.D. clinics who handle infected patients and touch the clinic knobs day in and day out don't pick up disease from such contacts or from the environment.

Nor will lack of cleanliness or poor personal hygiene, by themselves, ever lead to venereal disease. It requires the presence of micro-organisms, usually introduced into the body from another person harboring them. An individual cannot develop these infections on his or her own—they require partnership. A non-infected couple, limiting their sex life to each other, will not acquire a sexually transmitted disease. When someone with such an ailment tells a physician that this has been the case, somebody's not telling the truth, unless there has been a reactivation of an old and dormant infection.

Curing S.T.D.s

Aside from AIDS and herpes, the probability of curing an S.T.D. by medication is excellent. It is more difficult in those instances where the infection is caused by a virus. We still don't have very effective antibiotics against viruses. But even in the case of a non-viral infection, if an S.T.D. has gone untreated for some time, a cure can be effected but organs or tissues which have already been severely damaged may be beyond repair. *That's why it's important to seek early treatment if you have reason to suspect an infection.* Occasionally, one may luck out and have an S.T.D. that will ultimately cure itself—but you can't count on it.

Even for the most common S.T.D.s, *self*-treatment is not advisable and can frequently be dangerous. To prevent more serious effects on the body, proper medical care is essential. The reason for this is that the treatment is not the same for different individuals, at different stages of the disease, or for different complications.

A Global Epidemic

The new S.T.D.s are not restricted to any special part of the world. Because we're living in an age of constant global travel, which makes possible sexual relations between people hailing from different countries, no sexually transmitted disease remains localized for very long. One cannot safely assume that a sex partner in Paris or Sydney is less likely to have an infection than one in Peoria or San Francisco.

A Global Epidemic

The new S.T.D.s are not restricted to any special part of the world. Because we're living in an age of constant global travel, which makes possible sexual relations between people hailing from different countries, no sexually transmitted disease remains localized for very long. One cannot safely assume that a sex partner in Paris or Sydney is less likely to have an infection than one in Peoria or San Francisco.

CHAPTER TWO

Herpes

Twenty years ago the average adult outside of the medical community had never heard of herpes. Today it's a common affliction and a household word, something most educated people are aware of, even if they themselves don't suffer from it.

The full name of this wretched ailment is herpes simplex. It is one of the more common sexually transmitted diseases and has, despite progress in treatment, reached epidemic proportions. In its S.T.D. context, we speak of herpes genitalis, which means herpes around the genital areas. Both men and women can have herpes—in fact, it often ping-pongs back and forth between the partners in a heterosexual relationship. This is not to say that only heterosexuals get it—not so. Homosexuals, too, get herpes. Often.

What It Is And How You Get It

The word herpes stems from the Greek word "to creep" and it's an illness that's been around for almost as long as we have medical records. The Roman Emperor Tiberius tried to wipe out the disease by making kissing illegal but he failed, as have others since then, who have tried everything from no kissing to no sexual intercourse. Sexual abstinence might prevent a herpes sufferer from passing along the disease, but it will not cure one who is already infected.

Herpes is caused by a virus similar to the one that causes what is commonly referred to as "cold sores" or "fever blisters" around the mouth. It's an infection that is easily transmitted from the skin of one person to another if that person is susceptible. Some people are highly prone to it, while others enjoy greater resistance to this particular organism. Among those who are susceptible, contact with someone who has genital herpes can lead to quick and painful eruptions. Those who are little affected by herpes can still transmit the infection, even if they themselves experience only a minor eruption. The rate at which herpes occurs is about equal for men and women, and the physical and psychological distress it can produce is also about equal for both sexes.

The virus which usually causes fever blisters or cold sores on the lips is known as herpes simplex virus Type I. Such an outbreak on the skin is originally acquired through contact—but not necessarily sexual contact—and it can appear at any age, even in small children. After initial outbreak, and once it's in the system, it can be triggered by a number of factors: a cold, exposure to the sun, menstrual periods, and circumstances which lessen one's resistance. Both physical and mental stress can act as triggering agents, but the virus has to be there in the first place for a new eruption to appear.

Herpes simplex Type II is the one that causes skin eruptions below the belt, principally around the genitals. They can also occur on the thighs, on the buttocks, on the clitoris, in the anal area, or anywhere else on the skin. In the past, herpes on this part of the body was almost always Type II, but of late we see both types there. Only rarely do we see Type II on the face, but it does occur. So, to some degree, both types can now be found in either area.

Between outbreaks, the herpes hasn't been cured, it's merely dormant. During such remissions the viruses lodge in nerve cells near the lower spinal cord where they can remain for the life of the infected person even though he or she may rarely, if ever, experience another overt bout with the disease.

Common Symptoms And Diagnosis

A typical eruption of herpes looks like a cluster of little blisters on a reddened area of the skin. The blisters eventually break and form small sores. If there are several of them, they can fuse into one large ulcer which is referred to medically as a superficial "herpetic lesion."

The blisters, which can be very painful, erupt from two to ten days after contact with the virus. When they burst, millions of infectious virus particles are discharged. These viruses multiply very rapidly within the cells, and though the sores will heal within a week to ten days, the viruses, as I mentioned, remain in the body.

The pain which accompanies herpes lesions is one way in which they differ from the sores of syphilis, which don't hurt. During a herpes outbreak, particularly during the first outbreak, the lymph nodes in that area of the body, frequently in the groin, often become swollen and painful as well.

The first eruption of herpes can also be accompanied by a slight fever and flu-like symptoms. While fever is less common during subsequent eruptions, people often complain of general malaise and tiredness during the early stages of the outbreak. Some people who have frequent eruptions know a day or two in advance of their appearance that such an outbreak is on the way. During this period, usually twenty-four to forty-eight hours before an outbreak, there are mild and vague symptoms known as a prodrome and characterized by a feeling of discomfort at the site, sometimes by a slight pain or itching. However, it is possible for a herpes sufferer to experience the prodrome without it being followed by an eruption. When the eruption does occur, the degree of discomfort varies considerably; some people have excruciating pain, others are hardly aware of the outbreak, experiencing nothing more than mild discomfort.

Herpes simplex is one of the S.T.D.s that can usually be diagnosed by its characteristic appearance alone, provided one is trained in this field. Other factors confirm the diagnosis: the pain or discomfort, possible swelling of the lymph nodes, the fact that recurrences are usually in the same spot, and the general feeling of malaise.

However, not all superficial ulcers in the genital region are herpes. Reaching a diagnosis of herpes means eliminating the possibility of syphilis, in which the lesion may bear some resemblance to the herpes eruption. In the case of the syphilitic chancre there is a harder base, the lesion is not painful, it lasts longer, and it doesn't recur. But, since not all eruptions look as precisely characteristic as they should, we rely on lab tests to help distinguish one from the other. Where there is any doubt, cultures for the herpes virus can be done; and if the eruption is on the cervix, a Pap test (see page 186) can aid in the diagnosis. The Darkfield Test, discussed in the chapter on syphilis, can—if negative—usually rule out early syphilis. Of course, on rare occasions, herpes and syphilis infections can coexist.

Most Common Sites for Herpes

The herpes virus isn't choosey—an eruption can appear just about anywhere on the skin and on mucous membranes. It can be inside the vagina, on the cervix, on the finger—even on the eyeball or in the throat, or anywhere else for that matter. In men, the eruptions most commonly appear on the penis; in women, most often on the labia. But eruptions on the skin *near* the genitals—such as on the thighs and buttocks—are also common.

While herpes can occur in the mouth, the sores should not be confused with canker sores, which are quite painful but harmless, and due to a different virus. Since in herpes, in the early stages at least, several small, distinct blisters can be seen, a physician can usually tell the difference between the two ailments by their appearance.

Herpes And Kissing

You can transmit a virus with any body contact, and kissing is no exception, if the kissee is susceptible to the infection. But then, cold sores on the face are visible, and one would expect that someone experiencing a bout of facial herpes would refrain, temporarily, from kissing anyone. The problem, however, is that the virus can be transmitted several days before the eruption actually becomes evident, during the "shedding" period, which lasts from the onset of the prodrome to after the blisters have erupted. This is the most contagious period of the cycle, during which time sexual contact is not advisable.

Greeting casual acquaintances with a kiss on the mouth, or smoking a communal cigarette, much in vogue with people who use marijuana, are practices that have contributed to the spread of the herpes epidemic.

Recurrence: The Herpes Cycle

The frequency with which herpes will recur after the initial incident varies considerably from person to person. Some people have eruptions twice a month, or more often, with little time between the end of one outbreak and the beginning of another. Needless to say, this can wreak havoc with their sex life. Others, however, may have outbreaks as infrequently as once or twice a year. There are still others who suffer an episode of herpes and are never troubled by it again. What determines the frequency of recurrences is not the virus but an individual's susceptibility to it. The same infection in the source person and in someone he or she subsequently infects may have a totally different course—highly troublesome in one of the persons involved, barely perceptible in the other.

Those who have minimal symptoms and those who are totally asymptomatic can be silent carriers who are unaware that they are infected with herpes. They may pass it along in all innocence. Approximately half of all herpes victims show no symptoms or, at most, show them only during the initial outbreak.

Other Herpes-Related Infections

Members of the herpes virus family come in many varieties but most of them are non-infectious in humans. Type I and Type II are close relatives within the herpes simplex family. But this group also encompasses other members including the chicken pox virus, which causes herpes zoster (shingles) in adults; and another whose name crops up frequently these days, called cytomegalovirus. Because shingles is not a sexually transmitted disease (though it can be a complication of AIDS) I will not discuss it in this book.

Cytomegalovirus not only causes disease in susceptible adults (where it is not apparent on the skin and can have a great variety of manifestations, including fever), but it occasionally strikes newborn infants. Another virus that belongs to this herpes group is the one that causes infectious mononucleosis, called the Epstein-Barr virus. In all of these related infections, recurrences rarely happen. There is no cross-immunity between any of them, however, or with the virus of genital herpes. In other words, you can have mononucleosis or shingles and probably never get that ailment again, but the immunity you acquired against them will not prevent you from getting herpes progenitalis.

Women in their child-bearing years should also be aware that during pregnancy, herpes can be transmitted to the fetus or to the infant during birth. This is a relatively rare occurrence. But considering how widespread herpes infections are today, the existence of herpes should be mentioned to one's obstetrician even if no eruption is currently present. It poses a problem for the physician, who must make the decision whether to perform a Caesarian section to protect the newborn from direct contact with the herpes site, or whether to permit normal birth. It is a question of calculating one risk against another. Occasionally, a woman may be unaware that she has a herpes genitalis infection and it escapes prenatal detection by the physician. If an infant is infected, the infection is potentially serious because the newborn has little or no immunity against this virus. Annually, about two hundred infants are born with herpes simplex and approximately twenty-five percent of them die.

There has of late been much concern about the possibility that women suffering from herpes in the genital area run an increased risk of developing cervical cancer. As of now, the evidence produced by research is neither sufficient nor convincing enough to justify worry about this possibility in women who have bouts of herpes. (Actually, another virus, the human papilloma virus—HPV—appears to be more involved in causing a variety of genital cancers in both men and women.) However, a Pap test every year (see page 186), particularly for women who are middle-aged or older, is a good idea. In the child-bearing years, women who have herpes should also have routine Pap tests, if only to give them peace of mind when the findings regarding cancer of the cervix are negative.

Herpes And Sexual Activity

If an active herpes is on the penis or on the labia, it can be transmitted by intercourse; if on the mouth, it can be transmitted by kissing or oral sex; if in the rectal area, by anal intercourse. But even aside from contagion, which should be sufficient to deter most people from having intercourse during the infectious period, herpes can interfere with sexual activity because of discomfort. During this infectious stage (from the onset of the prodrome until after the blisters have finished shedding and become dry), the use of a condom can be helpful and make abstinence unnecessary. The condom is helpful regardless of whether it's a man or a woman who is experiencing the outbreak, provided the herpes cluster is in the path of the penis, or on it.

There are other precautions which can be taken since the infected lesions shed herpes viruses. If you are experiencing an outbreak and don't want to abstain from intercourse, avoid letting the infected area touch your partner. You can cover the lesions with some dry, physical barrier such as undershorts or pajamas. And, of course, you need not refrain from touching, caressing, and sexual arousal. Such restrictions are unnecessary if you exercise care to see that the lesion doesn't touch the other person. Since a woman can usually see or feel a labial lesion, she will usually know which part of her body should be kept away from her mate. These methods are not foolproof since lesions may be contagious even when hidden or minimal.

Treatment Of Herpes: Some Tips

I said at the beginning of this chapter that herpes has reached epidemic proportions. Estimates on how many suffer from this disease range from five to fifteen million, and the Centers for Disease Control (CDC), the U.S. government agency in Atlanta which tracks contagious diseases, has said that the figure might actually be as high as twenty million. It is estimated that as many as half a million new cases develop each year.

Social, demographic and behavioral changes within the U.S. population during the '70s and the early '80s have placed an increased proportion of our population at risk for sexually transmitted disease. During those years, herpes was one of the S.T.D.s that experienced dramatic growth. While the reported data about this disease can be assumed to reveal only the tip of the iceberg, certain figures will give you a clue to the speed with which the epidemic has escalated. The CDC did a study of the herpes situation from 1969 to 1979. Although data are far from complete, they showed that in 1969 there were 29,560 recorded consultations with physicians for genital herpes. In 1979, that number had gone to 260,890. By the mid-'80s, this number had increased to 450,000, with the incidence about the same in men and women, adults twenty to thirty years of age accounting for the largest proportion of cases.

Genital herpes increased uniformly in all regions of the U.S. The surveys mentioned do not, of course, include those infected who experience only minor or minimal symptoms, even though such cases can transmit the infection. Obviously, the figures would be considerably higher if all such consultations were reported—which they aren't, because many patients seek help from outpatient departments of community hospitals and from private physicians who do not always report these patient visits.

Because the disease is so widespread, a great deal of research is being carried out in this field in the hope that a useful remedy, if not a cure, might be developed. One product, called Acyclovir (Zovirax), in the form of an ointment, has been approved by the Food & Drug Administration (FDA) for use when prescribed by a physician. This ointment should be applied four to six times a day. Its manufacturer does not claim it to be a cure; it relieves pain and itching and shortens the duration of the outbreak. It is most effective when used at the time of the initial infection. It does not prevent recurrences and it is much less effective if used only in outbreaks that occur *after* the initial episode.

The same company produces an oral (tablet) form of this drug, which may be somewhat more effective than the ointment. Acyclovir tablets, too, reduce the symptoms of first episodes of herpes and shorten the healing time. The period of viral shedding is also reduced. However, it does not have much influence on the frequency of recurrences. While opinions are divided, it appears to be useful mostly to those with many recurrences and whose lives are adversely affected by such frequent and severe outbreaks. For infrequent and mild recurrences, its superiority over the ointment has not been fully established. Even when taking this oral medication, sexual intercourse should be avoided until the lesions are completely healed.

While Acyclovir succeeds in shortening the contagious period by a day or two, it does not work on everyone. Still, the drug shows that progress is being made and herpes sufferers have cause to be hopeful about further advances toward treatment and cure. Meanwhile, should Acyclovir as an ointment or in tablet form prove helpful in your particular case, you will at least be able to shorten the duration of each episode.

Acyclovir is also produced for intravenous use, but it is a potent drug that at this time can be administered only in hospitals. It is reserved for newborn infants with herpes who might otherwise die, for cases of encephalitis, and for cancer patients getting chemotherapy, in whom a herpes infection threatens to attack vital organs. Since life-threatening infections in infants are being treated quite successfully with these intravenous injections, the door is open to further research.

There are also a number of soothing preparations which some herpes sufferers find helpful. Covering the sores with a bland ointment such as sterile petroleum jelly (vaseline) will lessen friction against underwear and will cut down on the chance of a super-infection with another micro-organism. If the sore is near the urethra, it reduces the scalding sensation felt when urinating. *Cortisone ointments should not be used, as they can aggravate herpes.*

If you have herpes, it's a good idea to wear cotton underwear, rather than synthetics, because cotton absorbs moisture—the area should be kept as dry as possible. You should also avoid tight jeans or any tight clothing which might create friction in the area of the outbreak. Keeping the affected area dry is, as I said, advisable. After a shower or a bath, the area should be patted dry without friction. Don't rub it with your towel. Prolonged "sitzbaths" are not recommended. They provide temporary relief, but they can lead to maceration (undue softening) of the surrounding skin and invite the spreading of the clusters.

The Psychological Aspects Of Herpes

Painful as are the physical symptoms of herpes, many afflicted with this infection consider the psychological effects to be equally painful, or worse. Those who contracted herpes during an extramarital liaison have strong feelings of guilt and shame, and there are many reports that the disease has caused the breakup of marriages and other relationships. Upon learning that they have contracted herpes, people often experience a feeling of disbelief that is usually followed by anger at the person from whom the victim got it.

One of the major problems faced by herpes sufferers is whether or not to tell their sexual partners that they have the infection. Since each person's relationship with another is highly individual, there is obviously no single answer to this distressing problem.

Apart from progress being made in treating herpes with drugs, there is another encouraging fact. Over the years, the attacks get fewer and are spaced further apart. In many people, the herpes virulence seems to exhaust itself after three to five years, and even when there are recurrences, they come with less frequency and are less severe. Furthermore, since in many people the episodes are triggered by psychological factors, these are often controllable, either through psychiatric help or by psychotherapeutic drugs.

As far as treatment for herpes is concerned, the future looks promising. And if you're reading this chapter and *don't* have herpes (or any other S.T.D., for that matter) perhaps you will want to conclude that it's a good idea to know someone intimately on other levels before committing yourself to a sexual relationship. Even though the public scare over herpes that existed in the early '80s has been eclipsed by the alarm over AIDS, herpes remains a major public health problem.

CHAPTER THREE

Non-Gonococcal Urethritis

The symptoms of non-gonococcal urethritis are not unlike those of gonorrhea: a discharge from the urethra, seen at the tip of the penis, often combined with some burning and an urge to urinate frequently. Years ago, when a man had such symptoms and could associate them with a recent sexual contact, it was assumed that he had gonorrhea. But it has recently become evident that a majority of such cases are actually caused by a variety of *other* micro-organisms.

We used to believe that such micro-organisms, though troublesome, were relatively harmless. Over the years, however, we've learned that, if untreated, they can do as much harm, sometimes *more* harm, than a gonococcal infection. They can creep up the urethra and affect organs of the upper genital tract, such as the prostate; and they can even affect distant organs like the liver, the eyes, and the joints.

Though similar to the symptoms of gonorrhea, those in non-gonococcal urethritis are usually milder. Gonorrhea, however, can also be quite mild at times, thus it's not possible to make a diagnostic distinction between the two merely on the basis of a patient's complaints. A microscopic examination and/or cultures are required to tell one from the other. One difference between the two types of infection is that the incubation time for non-gonococcal infections is usually much longer than the two-to-five days for gonorrhea—it can take anywhere from seven to twenty-eight days. But none of this is absolute. There are exceptions.

Organisms Causing Non-Gonococcal Urethritis

The micro-organism most frequently found in this infection is the chlamydia (trachomatis), which is neither a bacterium nor a virus. (Chlamydial infections are discussed in more detail in Chapter 4.) This organism accounts for only a third to half of all the cases of non-gonococcal urethritis.

There are a variety of others that can be responsible for this ailment. One group found occasionally is known as mycoplasm, discussed in Chapter 10, the chapter on *Other Sexually Transmissible Diseases*. In many cases it simply isn't known what produces the symptoms. Because of difficulty in pinning down the causative agent, the group of infections is lumped together under the broad and general name of non-gonococcal urethritis. This is a non-commital term that more or less implies that it's not possible to be precise in the diagnosis.

In addition to the chlamydia and the mycoplasms, of which ureaplasma urealyticum is one, non-gonococcal urethritis can also be caused by trichomonas, a common infection in the female genital tract; and by candida, a fungal type of infection also found frequently in the vagina, which is occasionally transmissible to the male during intercourse. But this does not occur very often. Even herpes can cause urethritis, as can bacteria like the coliforms, which are common in the bowel. These bacteria have no reason to be in the male urethra, but anal intercourse will sometimes cause an inappropriate transfer of site.

Not infrequently, a patient may have N.G.U. *and* gonorrhea at the same time.

Complications Due To Non-Gonococcal Urethritis

Because this disease category comprises a number of different types of infections, the symptoms can also vary greatly. A man can be infected and be unaware of it because he has no symptoms. He might learn of his infection if his sex partner has an infection which recurs despite successful treatment. This would direct attention to an infected but asymptomatic lover.

If untreated (usually because a man is unaware he has it) it's possible to develop what are called "ascending" infections: the causing organisms creep along the genital path, and, as I said above, infect other organs. This could cause a chronic ache in the region of the prostate or testicles; could cause swelling; and could, untreated, lead to sterility. Furthermore, if a man with non-gonococcal urethritis infects a woman, she can develop a different set of ailments, including cervicitis (an inflammation of the tip of the womb) and P.I.D., *Pelvic Inflammatory Disease,* discussed in detail in Chapter 6.

Diagnosis And Treatment

This diagnosis is usually made by exclusion. If there are symptoms of urethritis, and gonococci cannot be found either on a stained smear or in a culture, then it's obviously non-gonococcal urethritis. Cultures for other organisms can then be done—but such tests are not usually performed because they're time-consuming and they can involve considerable cost. Each test is eight to ten times as expensive as the test for gonococci and one might do many such tests and still find nothing.

In cases of this sort, therefore, it's quicker, simpler, and more in the interest of the patient's health to treat the urethritis on the basis of the physician's impression of what it is. Of course, in unusual cases and in persistent ones, the doctor will usually go ahead with the complex diagnostic procedures to try and identify the specific causative agent.

Since it's not always known which agent is responsible for the urethritis, it's generally treated with antibiotics that have a broad range of effectiveness against the most likely causes. These antibiotics are the tetracyclines. It usually takes a longer course of treatment to cure a non-gonococcal infection than to cure gonorrhea—at least twice as long, which would make it about eight to ten days. Often, a third treatment course with the same medication has to be added. There are other antibiotics, such as the erythromycin group of drugs, that are also effective and, if response is poor, there are still other alternative drugs that can be prescribed.

Preventing Recurrences

Non-gonococcal urethritis likes to return. In such cases, treatment may be repeated for a longer period of time; or a different antibiotic might be prescribed. In very persistent cases, with frequent recurring bouts, a search might be initiated to determine what is causing the repetition.

A most important factor in preventing recurrences is to treat one's steady sex partner even if that person is without symptoms. As with other sexually transmitted infections, one person can be greatly affected while another, harboring the same organism, may be entirely asymptomatic. Use of a condom will greatly reduce the likelihood of future infections.

CHAPTER FOUR

Chlamydial Infections

Chances are that if you're old enough to have been sexually active ten years ago, you never heard of chlamydia (pronounced kla-mid-ia) at that time. You may not have heard of it five years ago. Today, sexually active men and women who are not monogamous hear of chlamydia from friends, acquaintances, relatives, and physicians. Not that everyone walks around talking about chlamydia—obviously this is not a topic of conversation at your average dinner table. But this infection is so common—it is, in fact, far more common than gonorrhea—that one would have to be quite isolated to be unaware of its existence.

What It Is And How It Differs From Gonorrhea

The proper name of the micro-organism that causes this S.T.D. is chlamydia trachomatis. For almost a century, chlamydia has been known to medicine as producing a widely prevalent disease in countries of low hygienic standards. That disease has been known as trachoma. It is an infection of the conjunctivae, the pinkish mucosa lining that is part of the eyeball. This eye disease is a serious one affecting both children and adults; if untreated, it can gradually lead to blindness. Globally speaking, it is the most frequent cause of blindness.

However, in countries such as ours, with advanced standards of hygiene, we rarely see trachoma. Yet here at home, chlamydial infections have developed into a type of sexually transmitted disease that we see in our medical offices and clinics every day. The number of cases has, in fact, quadrupled in the last ten years.

The organism in this disease is much smaller than the gonococcus, which is the one that causes gonorrhea, and it is difficult to grow in cultures outside the body because it develops and multiplies only in live cells. The gonococcus is, as the name tells us, a coccus, which means a dot-shaped organism. The chlamydia trachomatis and the gonococcus are unrelated—but they can produce a very similar disease picture. So similar are they, in fact, that even an experienced clinician often cannot tell the symptoms of one from the other without the help of a laboratory.

Symptoms Produced By Chlamydia

In developed countries, such as the U.S., chlamydial infection of the eyes is almost always due to a secondary spread from the genitals, if they are infected. But it can also be found in the eyes of newborn infants if the mother has a chlamydial infection of the birth canal.

The principal symptoms produced by the chlamydia are those of non-gonococcal urethritis discussed in the previous chapter. You will recall that these symptoms are often much like those in gonorrhea: a whitish discharge from the penis, the urge to urinate frequently, and some burning sensation in men. Most women with chlamydia have no symptoms at all; or at most, a slight discharge and possibly a frequent desire to urinate. Because the symptoms in women are mild or nonexistent, they are less likely to be treated when the infection is new. This is unfortunate because the infection gets a chance to move upwards where it can infect the Fallopian tubes, creating a Pelvic Inflammatory Disease (P.I.D.) known as salpingitis. Since it's the tubes that carry the eggs from the ovaries to the uterus, infertility can result if the tubes become blocked. Sometimes, scars on the tubes will hold an egg there, and should it become fertilized, an ectopic pregnancy (tubal pregnancy) may result. Should it begin to develop and cause the tube to rupture, a serious medical emergency might exist. Unfortunately, we have seen more ectopic pregnancies in recent years because of the considerable increase in cases of Pelvic Inflammatory Disease.

Chlamydia can produce other symptoms as well: the symptoms of prostatitis (an inflammation of the prostate gland); epididymitis (an inflammation of the organ that hugs the testicles); proctitis (an inflammation of the anal canal); and P.I.D. in women, usually characterized by lower abdominal pain. I'll discuss this in detail in the next chapter. Chlamydia can even cause pain around the liver. And, as I said, it can cause conjunctivitis. It can also cause pneumonia in the newborn.

Symptomatic chlamydial infections are now three times more common than gonorrhea—and possibly even more than that. One of the reasons for this is that we don't have simple lab tests such as we have for gonorrhea, so that many people go undiagnosed. If symptomless, they are unaware that they have the disease and become carriers—people who transmit the disease without knowing it.

There is a relatively new development, for which we don't have an exact explanation. Among college students, chlamydial infections are as much as ten times more common than gonococcal infections. In fact, many students who think they have gonorrhea actually have other types of infections of which chlamydia is but one. Statistically, we do know that gonorrhea is not passed around as much among the well-educated and well-read—so there is less of it on campus than in the lower socio-economic strata.

Absence Of Symptoms

The symptom-free carrier may harbor this disease for a long period of time, perhaps for years, without suffering any personal ill-effects. However, since such people give the disease to others, treatment is necessary if the organism is found in a test. Furthermore, a person without symptoms may actually develop serious complications. The most common of the serious complications is, of course, sterility.

It's easy to see what a problem is created by symptomless carriers. A sex partner may become infected, have some complaints, go for treatment, get cured, and then promptly be reinfected again unless the seemingly unaffected partner gets treatment, too. For this reason, someone being treated for chlamydia, as for the more traditional venereal diseases, is always urged to have his or her partner come in for treatment.

Other Fertility Problems

Chlamydia can do more than cause a woman's Fallopian tubes to become blocked. It can also affect the lining of the womb, leading to premature birth, stillbirth, or neo-natal death. This is not to say that, given such an infection in a woman, all these things—or *any* of them—are definitely going to occur. In the majority of cases, even a woman with an undiagnosed case of chlamydia is capable of becoming pregnant and having a normal delivery. The complications of chlamydia are things which can and do occur—but in a minority of cases.

Other Diseases Produced By This Organism

There are some species of chlamydia, the organism, that are distant cousins to the one that causes a sexually transmitted disease. One of these is psittacosis, a common disease among birds, which occasionally affects people who feed birds (particularly parakeets) or are otherwise in contact with them. Lymphogranuloma venereum, another human sexually transmitted disease, is also caused by an agent that's in the chlamydia family. This is not a common S.T.D. and not one that you need to worry about.

Tests And Treatment For Chlamydia

A variety of tests for chlamydia do exist but, unfortunately, the only reliable one at this time is the tissue culture method. I say "unfortunate" because this method takes time. It's not only slow, but the test is not available in many places; and when it is available, it's costly. Virtually no private physician's office or health department clinic is equipped to do a culture for chlamydia. They are ordinarily done in virology labs or by some private laboratories. But if every suspected case of chlamydia were to be diagnosed by that method, then there would not be enough labs to do all the required cultures.

Consequently, chlamydia is usually diagnosed by eliminating what the infection is *not*. If it is *not* gonorrhea and the symptoms are those of chlamydia, the infection will usually be diagnosed as "non-gonococcal" urethritis, or "non-specific" urethritis, or inflammation of the cervix, etc. Obviously, it's in the best interest of the patient to be treated promptly, particularly where there are annoying or painful symptoms. So, for the most part, clinicians treat for the presence of a chlamydial infection if there is reasonable suspicion that it exists. This state of affairs in terms of diagnosis is likely to change as we develop better testing methods for chlamydia.

The treatment of a chlamydial infection consists in taking what is called a broad-spectrum antibiotic; in particular, a tetracycline. Generally speaking (as always, there are exceptions) it takes considerably longer for a treatment course to cure a chlamydial infection than to achieve a cure for gonorrhea. It may take seven days to eradicate chlamydia, and the amount of medication, which is taken daily, can usually be smaller than that used for gonorrhea. (This was discussed more specifically in the preceding chapter, when I talked about non-gonococcal urethritis.) During a pregnancy, erythromycin is given instead of tetracyclines.

One does not develop an immunity to either a chlamydial infection or to gonorrhea, so recurrences do occur. Unfortunately, that means if the natural disease does not leave any future resistance against the infection, a vaccine cannot be better in producing immunity than the disease itself. Vaccines against these infections are, therefore, unlikely to be developed, or to be effective. New infections can be acquired after an old one is cured—or, an old infection that left a few organisms lurking in some organ insufficiently affected by antibiotics, can cause the disease to flare up again. In particular, this may happen if the prostate was affected.

As with all S.T.D.s, some basic advice applies. Monogamy with a monogamous partner is, of course, the best protection against infection. The condom, which is not too popular with men, is another protection. Beyond these two, the best way to discourage infection is to know something about the habits and life style of the person you're going to get involved with sexually. And get medical attention if you have symptoms of any S.T.D.—or reason to believe that someone you slept with has, or had, such an infection.

CHAPTER FIVE

Vaginitis

Specific and Non-specific

Vaginitis is an irritation or inflammation of the vagina.

This is a general term which comprises those disorders that are due to sexually transmitted infections as well as others which are not. Vaginitis can produce discomfort or pain and is often characterized by a discharge—sometimes slight, sometimes heavy.

These disorders are not necessarily started by infections. There is also a condition known as "chemical vaginitis," usually induced by improper douching. Women occasionally use inappropriate substances in their douche water— such as bicarbonate of soda, hydrogen peroxide, and even Lysol—that can injure the mucous membrane of the vaginal wall and produce a chronic, painful irritation. Sometimes a commercial douche preparation can be harmful if a woman happens to be hyper-sensitive to the substance. In other instances, women who assume that "if a little bit is good, a lot is even better" will use too high a concentration of an otherwise innocuous douching preparation. This can result in a chemical vaginitis. And then there are those women who feel the first signs of vaginal irritation and douche even more, with higher concentrations of the douching substance. Frequently, this will only aggravate the condition.

You will find more on the subject of douching in my chapter on that subject (Chapter 12, pp. 111 to 115). I will only add here that the persistent doucher with chronic vaginitis should refrain from all douching for several weeks to find out whether this, by itself, will produce a cure. Often, it will.

Difference Between Specific And Non-Specific Vaginitis

Vaginitis is most often produced by micro-organisms that can be identified on microscopic examination or by culturing some material taken from the vaginal wall. There are three types of micro-organisms that are most often the culprits, and they are common enough to be well known. They are monilia, trichomonas and gardnerella vaginalis, all discussed below. A clinician will usually search for these and if one is found, the vaginitis is "specific."

If examination does not reveal one of these three causative organisms, or any other invading germ, but the signs of vaginitis are real nonetheless, then the term "non-specific vaginitis" is tagged to the complaint. In other words, it means that the inflammation is present but we are not sure what has caused it.

Monilia is also known as candida albicans and the disease it produces is called moniliasis, or thrush. All three organisms—monilia, trichomonas, and gardnerella vaginalis—

can be sexually transmitted, but are not necessarily so. They are extremely common and often inhabit the vagina without causing any disorder or symptom. They just live there, in harmony with the environment. Depending upon individual circumstances, however, there can be an overgrowth of such micro-organisms that can then lead to vaginitis.

Moniliasis, Also Known As Thrush

As I said, moniliasis is one of the most common infections of the vagina and, though it is sexually transmissible, it is *not* a venereal disease. It's caused by a yeast-like organism, usually non-virulent, that belongs to the fungus family. Just as ringworm thrives on moist skin, so does monilia flourish on the moist lining of the vagina. While this is almost always a harmless infection, it can be a nuisance because it can produce an unsightly sort of white, thickish discharge.

This organism likes sweets, so it's partial to diabetics and others who have sugar in their urine. It also flourishes during pregnancy and in persons who take certain antibiotics (such as tetracyclines) for prolonged periods of time. But it's not limited to people in those categories—it's quite common in individuals who are otherwise perfectly healthy.

A man's genitals may also be infected with monilia, although this is relatively rare. When it occurs, it usually affects the skin at the tip of the penis and can make it appear red, raw, or "weeping." Since thrush likes warm, moist environments, it is more likely to be found in men who are not circumcised. Some men are carriers—they harbor the monilia organisms, but the lack of symptoms makes them unaware of their presence. Men who are carriers can transmit the organism during intercourse.

Treatment For Moniliasis

Minor cases of this infection are common, cause no discomfort, and do not require treatment. However, if annoying symptoms develop, the ailment should be treated by a physician. Antibiotics exist which are effective in clearing up the infection but you need a prescription to get such drugs. An older remedy that is also quite effective and available without prescription is gentian-violet, a dye that is introduced into the vagina either in vaginal suppositories or jellies. This method is a bit messy and leaves a telltale stain for quite a while. Gentian-violet requires no prescription.

Fungal antibiotics commonly prescribed are Miconazole or Clotrimazole (Lotrimin). They are available as cream or tablets (100, 200, and 500 mg). Depending on the strength of the preparation, they are used vaginally for two to seven days.

Nystatin is another fungal antibiotic available in tablet form. One tablet intra-vaginally, daily for two weeks, usually clears up the infection. All of these are prescription drugs.

Trichomoniasis

Trichomoniasis (pronounced trick-o-moan-i-asis) is an infection with trichomonas, which are larger than bacteria and can easily be seen under a microscope as they move around, propelled by a whip-like movement that enables them to travel rapidly. They, too, are common; in fact, they are to be found in one-third of all women. When they're present in small numbers, they usually cause little or no trouble and are just as well left alone. But their overgrowth (some people are more susceptible to such an overgrowth than are others) can produce disturbing symptoms which might include itching, a scalding sensation, and an irritating discharge with a characteristic odor to it. Such cases do, of course, require proper diagnosis and treatment.

As with moniliasis, men can be carriers of trichomoniasis and can transmit the infection even though they, themselves, usually have no symptoms. It's difficult to determine whether or not a man is infected with trichomonas. Sometimes the disease will produce a prostatitis (inflammation of the prostate gland) or urethritis (inflammation of the urethra). But since a man may carry the infection and not have any symptoms, it's always advisable when a woman is being treated for a trichomonas infection that her steady partner, if she has one, be treated as well, and at the same time. Otherwise, the infection can be ping-ponged back and forth.

Treatment For Trichomoniasis

Trichomonas are quite sensitive to a chemical called Metronidazole, which is a prescription drug taken orally. These tablets, taken over a period of one to seven days, can terminate an infection with trichomonas. Of course, as I said, if a woman has a steady sex partner, he should be treated as well. If he is not treated, the woman could find herself right back where she started.

When resistance to treatment occurs it is not usually an *absolute* resistance. It means that a longer treatment course, or perhaps a larger dose of medication, will be required to achieve a cure. On rare occasions this organism does resist Metronidazole, but new, effective antibiotics will soon be available to treat this ailment. Incidentally, when taking medication for trichomoniasis, avoid alcoholic beverages. The two are incompatible.

Before treatment is initiated, a diagnosis should be confirmed by lab tests (either direct microscopic examination or a culture for trichomonas). In those rare instances when a treatment does fail, it's usually due to one of three things: the diagnosis was wrong; re-infection took place; or there may be a real, if uncommon, drug resistance by the micro-organisms.

One more point: even when a correct diagnosis of trichomoniasis has been made, this may not be the only cause of a vaginitis. The presence of trichomonas can mask the presence of chlamydia or gonorrhea, which often coexist with it.

Gardnerella As A Cause Of Vaginitis

Gardnerella vaginalis, formerly known by other names like haemophilus vaginalis and corynebacterium vaginale, is another common inhabitant of the vagina. Again, this organism can cause trouble through overgrowth, or it can live in the vagina peacefully, requiring no treatment. Organisms of this type—those which may produce disease symptoms or may create no problems at all—are known as "facultative pathogens." Their common characteristic is that they are capable of coexisting with other organisms in the vagina but will, in some individuals, under some circumstances, create trouble.

Gardnerella infections, when troublesome, can be treated with Metronidazole (Flagyl), the same drug used to treat trichomoniasis. However, gardnerella may also respond to treatment with ampicillin. It is less effective, but it can be used during pregnancy, when Metronidazole should not be used.

Non-Specific Vaginitis

As I mentioned at the beginning of this chapter, and as the name implies, non-specific vaginitis is an inflammation or irritation of the vagina (usually accompanied by symptoms such as itching or discharge), where the more common micro-organisms of vaginitis do not appear to be implicated and no specific causative agent can be isolated or identified.

I spoke earlier about the fact that the vaginal wall can be affected by douching with the wrong substances or with too-high concentrations of acceptable ones. These douching procedures can damage the mucosal lining of the vagina and make it more susceptible to a variety of organisms—some sexually transmitted, others not—to which it would normally be immune.

Sometimes other factors contribute to non-specific vaginitis. One of these is lowered resistance to infections, such as that caused by other, coexisting illnesses.

Any woman who suffers from recurrent non-specific vaginitis should have an annual Pap test done. (See Chapter 20, p. 183.) The reason for this is that women who have frequent or prolonged bouts of vaginitis are more likely to develop changes in the lining of the cervix (the tip of the womb) and it's advisable to determine the existence of such changes early, when it's easier to treat them.

CHAPTER SIX

P.I.D.

Pelvic Inflammatory Disease

The term Pelvic Inflammatory Disease, commonly referred to as P.I.D., includes a lot. In the simplest terms, it is an infection that has spread to a woman's tubes, or beyond, from the lower genital organs, either the vagina or the womb. But P.I.D. can affect more than the tubes. It can also spread to adjoining organs such as the ovaries; or to the peritoneum, which is the lining of the organs in the abdomen.

Of all the sexually acquired diseases in women, P.I.D. is the most common complication. It is estimated that close to a million cases of P.I.D. occur annually in this country.

Salpingitis And P.I.D.

Although the phrase P.I.D. includes a disease known as salpingitis, the latter is a narrower term. It means an inflammation of one or both Fallopian tubes, the pipes that carry the egg from the ovary to the womb. It is often difficult to distinguish one from the other because it is difficult to determine the limits of the spread without looking into the abdomen with a peritoneoscope, or without surgery. Therefore, the two expressions are used more or less interchangeably.

The Symptoms of P.I.D.

Symptoms may vary from slight discomfort in the lower abdomen, on one side or both, to severe pain in the same area, usually accompanied by a somewhat elevated or high temperature. In some cases there may be a medical history of recent infection with an S.T.D., or of intercourse with a new sex partner. However, by no means are all P.I.D.s the result of a sexually transmitted disease.

Most often, the onset of P.I.D. is five to ten days after a menstrual period. In addition to the pain, other symptoms—less characteristic of this disease—include a vaginal discharge, frequency of urination, nausea, bleeding between periods, pain during intercourse, and occasionally, vomiting. The determination as to whether or not the symptoms are those of P.I.D. rests with the examining physician, whose advice should be sought in any case when there might be even a remote possibility of such trouble.

Other Disorders Mistaken for P.I.D.

Many other illnesses have symptoms very similar to those of Pelvic Inflammatory Disease. These would include acute appendicitis, which can be difficult to differentiate from an inflammation of the right Fallopian tube; or an ectopic preg nancy, which is a medical emergency that occurs if an egg is implanted in a tube and begins to develop there. Ovarian cysts and tumors can also mimic the symptoms of P.I.D.

P.I.D. and Gonorrhea

Only about a third of P.I.D. cases are caused by the gonococcus. Thus, gonorrhea should by no means be thought of as the only culprit to blame for such an illness. The other two-thirds of P.I.D. cases are caused by chlamydia and a variety of other organisms. Any of these organisms can be found alone or in combination with others—in that case, they're called polymicrobial infections. A combination of the gonococcus and of chlamydia is common.

There are some differences in both the symptoms and the course of treatment for P.I.D.s caused by the gonococcus and by chlamydia, but even in this we find many variations. There are no clear-cut dividing lines. Generally speaking, however, one can say that P.I.D. caused by the gonococcus is what we call, in medical slang, a "hotter" disease. It is usually more acute, producing more symptoms, greater pain, and higher temperatures.

Chlamydial infections, on the other hand, maintain a lower profile. They tend to last longer and require longer courses of treatment. Despite the fact that they seem less acute—or maybe *because* of it—they can cause greater damage in the long run. This might include a closure of the tubes. As I mentioned, the function of the tubes is to transport eggs from the ovaries to their nesting place in the womb, so a closure can lead to infertility. However, both tubes would need to be closed for this to happen.

Other Causes of P.I.D.

As I said, a Pelvic Inflammatory Disease is not always caused by a sexually acquired disease. An infection can follow the presence of an intra-uterine device in the womb and can then spread to the tubes. P.I.D. may occasionally follow an abortion. As you will see later on in the chapter on *Douching*, frequent and vigorous douches can sweep some organisms from the vagina into the womb and even past it, into the tubes. This is particularly true if such douching is done around the time of the menses, when the cervical canal is open.

During pregnancy, P.I.D. is rare. In fact, should pain occur in the lower abdomen during pregnancy, particularly if it's accompanied by an elevated temperature or any of the other symptoms described above, it is more likely to be appendicitis than P.I.D.

Prompt diagnosis and treatment are important. If you are using an I.U.D. and have symptoms that could suggest P.I.D., you should see your gynecologist or clinician. If the symptoms are mild or vague, any nearby V.D. clinic can advise you what to do, or refer you to an appropriate physician. At the other extreme, in acute cases where there is considerable pain and fever, the emergency room of the nearest hospital is the best resource for immediate care.

The type and length of treatment depends on the individual situation. Once diagnosis of P.I.D. is made, we rely on antibiotics to control the infection. Since we don't usually know which germs are involved, we treat with tetracycline drugs, such as doxycycline, because they hit a wide target. They are effective on most of the micro-organisms that could be involved in a P.I.D. However, when a case is extremely acute, with high temperature and great pain, the infection is more likely to be gonococcal; and a high dose of penicillin may be given initially, usually in the hospital. Ordinarily, it isn't wise to wait for an answer from the laboratory as to which organisms are involved. It is more important to render prompt treatment so that the patient gets some relief and the chances of further spreading are curbed.

Even if an infection turns out to be gonococcal, it is almost impossible to determine whether other infecting agents are also involved. Therefore, many clinicians will treat with another group of antibiotics *after* the penicillin, or instead of it. These antibiotics include Cefoxitin, Clindamycin, and Gentamycin—sometimes a combination of these drugs.

Whether or not hospitalization is required in the case of P.I.D. depends on the severity of the infection and the intensity of the symptoms. Were every minor case of P.I.D. to be admitted to a hospital, they would soon account for the largest percentage of patients. On the other hand, when there is any doubt at all about the diagnosis, it is preferable to go into the hospital. As mentioned earlier, the symptoms of P.I.D. can easily be confused with a number of other medical problems— some of them, such as appendicitis, are potentially serious. However, where a patient is reasonable, intelligent, and able to comply with medical instructions—provided, of course, that the symptoms are moderate—treatment as an out-patient is to be preferred.

Untreated P.I.D.

As mentioned previously, when a Pelvic Inflammatory Disease goes untreated, the Fallopian tubes may become blocked, leading to infertility. Another possible consequence of failure to get treatment is that the infection can spread and lead to the development of an abcess, or of peritonitis, which can, at times, become a life-threatening emergency.

Depending on the organism that caused it, an untreated P.I.D. can also become a persistent source of infection and reinfection of one's sex partners. Partners should be referred for evaluation and, if necessary, for treatment. Sexual activity should be avoided until both partners are cured.

Unfortunately, attacks of P.I.D. do not provide immunity against future episodes. On the contrary, people who have had a Pelvic Inflammatory Disease are more likely to get it again should they have an S.T.D. This is true whether the primary infection is gonococcal or non-gonococcal.

CHAPTER SEVEN

Gonorrhea

Perhaps a book on the *new* sexually transmitted diseases might be expected to exclude such old familiar faces as gonorrhea and syphilis. Both of these are still very much with us but there *is* something new about these two diseases: a leveling off, even a slight decline in their incidence. This became noticeable in the last few years, due to a moderate cooling trend in the lifestyles among some groups, particularly in the gay community and among the well-educated. Unfortunately, no radical decline has taken place as yet. Besides, no solid book on S.T.D.s would be complete if it didn't talk about communicable diseases that probably afflict over two million persons annually, in this country alone.

The most widespread of the reportable S.T.D.s is gonorrhea, which is caused by bacteria called gonococci (pronounced *gon-o-cocky*).

If gonorrhea is not as old as the hills, then it is at least as old as the first hill dwellers. This disease has been described in the oldest existing medical reports as far back as Hippocrates, and even in the Bible. There are also some possible references to it in early Oriental writings and in ancient Egyptian prescriptions.

Its prevalence, of course, has varied through the ages. It has peaked during times of wars and other major upheavals. In the '70s and early '80s, many countries were again experiencing a peak in gonorrhea incidence. I suggested some reasons for this in the first chapter, where I talked about the increasing prevalence of S.T.D.s.

The "Clap" And Other Synonyms

There are a number of slang terms for gonorrhea. The "clap" is one. Another is the "drip" and once in a while you hear it referred to as "strain," "G.C.," or a "dose." There really isn't, in proper English, a pleasant sounding word for it, but then, it isn't a very pleasant ailment.

The Symptoms, If Any

First, let's separate the men from the women.

Most often, in two to five days after contact with an infected person, a man may show some noticeable symptoms— then again, he may not. An ordinary, common case of male gonorrhea runs something like this: No signs on the first, second, perhaps third day after infection. Then, but sometimes a little later on, some discomfort begins at the tip of the penis. Urinating may become quite painful and produce a burning sensation. There may also be an urge to urinate frequently.

This discomfort is soon followed by a discharge of pus, slight at first but rapidly increasing. For a typical case it is yellowish in color and different from the normal, thin, water-clear, mucous-like discharge that appears when sexually aroused.

However, not every abnormal discharge from the penis is gonorrhea. There are other infections, usually transmitted by sexual contact, called non-gonococcal urethritis, which I discussed in Chapter 3. As in gonorrhea, these can also be troublesome and sometimes are even more persistent. It's of some importance for a proper diagnosis to be made, because if the discharge is due to a non-gonococcal agent, it usually requires more time to achieve a cure.

Male Organs Affected By Gonorrhea

Most commonly, only the urethra is affected. This is the small channel running through the center of the penis. If treated in time, the disease may be limited to this organ. Occasionally, however, and particularly if not treated early, gonorrhea may move higher up in the urinary system and affect the prostate gland, an organ the size of a chestnut located at the bladder exit. Once the infection is imbedded there, getting rid of it is more difficult. If it moves still higher, it may produce an inflammation in the tube-shaped organs that transport the sperm from the testicles. Any inflammation there, or in the testicle itself, can often be cured medically without aftereffects. However, a blockage may develop that can lead to sterility and that may be irreversible.

The infection can also spread beyond the sex organs and urinary tract. In both men and women (and I'll go into more detail later about gonorrhea in women), the micro-organisms can also enter the blood stream and settle in organs far removed from where they originally entered the body. This may include the joints and the lining of the heart. It could also affect the skin by producing little lesions that resemble pimples. And it can produce a rather serious type of eye infection. It can also cause an inflammation of the lining of the liver and lead to symptoms resembling those of a gallbladder attack or disease. All these complications occur more frequently in women than in men.

Complications in remote organs are not as common in men because they are more likely to seek medical attention earlier in the course of the infection. As I previously pointed out, that's because they're more likely to have acute discomfort. Eighty-five percent of newly infected men will look for early medical advice, while about half of the infected women may, at first, be unaware of having an infection—despite the fact that they may experience some early, vague, and noncharacteristic symptoms.

Visible Signs Of Infection In Men

Signs of an infection are not *always* evident in men. However, in most cases—perhaps eight or nine cases out of ten—the signs are there, at least in early gonorrhea. But in one or two out of ten where they aren't, only a bacteriological examination with a smear or culture will enable a clinician to detect the infection. The reasons why some men show no symptoms, or few, are unknown. Some individuals have a little more resistance and show fewer signs, yet their infection is every bit as communicable as any other.

The small percentage of men who have no symptoms and no complaints constitute a big problem. Sometimes, suspicion is aroused that an infection may exist when the man learns that a person with whom he had sexual intimacy has become infected. Such "carriers" of the germ can often spread the disease to others without any awareness that they are doing so.

In case you're not familiar with the term "carrier," it means someone—and it can be either a man or a woman—who is infected, is liable to infect other persons, yet is not suffering from any noticeable signs of the illness. This may happen at four different stages: when infected but having no symptoms; before symptoms have developed (this is really called the incubation period and not a carrier stage); when an acute infection has subsided but has not been cured; or when an infection has been insufficiently treated so that it lingers on without outward manifestations. Actually, women are more often carriers than men.

Telltale Symptoms in Women

Women are often unaware of having gonorrhea in the early stages. There may be some mild burning or itching that may not inspire a quick visit to a medical facility. Even if there is a discharge, it might be moderate and go unnoticed. However, women who are infected frequently have urinary discomfort or a frequent urge to empty the bladder; these women usually surmise correctly that they need medical attention.

Gonorrhea, if untreated or mistreated, can lead to Pelvic Inflammatory Disease (P.I.D.). In a complicated infection— that is, one that has spread—there can be severe abdominal pain, which may indicate that the tubes have been affected. If the disease progresses, there is also a possibility of further spreading and of peritonitis, an inflammation of the abdominal lining.

However, urinary discomforts caused by various forms of cystitis are very common in women who do *not* have a venereal disease. This is part of the problem in today's epidemic—and the reason why tests are called for to determine what's what. Many non-venereal infections can cause symptoms similar to those in gonorrhea. In fact, many common troubles that women experience with their bladders and sex organs are *not* due to S.T.D.s. These include burning or itching when urinating, and a whitish discharge. Regardless of how moderate these symptoms may appear to be, anyone experiencing them should get medical attention.

Female Organs Affected By Gonorrhea

Any organ immediately adjacent to the vagina can be involved. Usually, it is the lining of the tip of the womb and the area around the urethra—the duct which carries urine away from the bladder. Infections can also take place in the rectum—and these are by no means rare. As with the organs around the vagina, a rectal infection may give little or no discomfort, and a woman may be unaware that she is infected. If the disease is permitted to spread, unchecked by treatment, it can also affect other organs, both distant from and adjoining the vagina. Rectal infections are not rare in women and in homosexual men.

Effect Of The Menstrual Cycle On Gonorrhea

Around the time of the menstrual period, gonorrhea tends to spread into the womb and past the womb into the tubes, causing inflammation and pain. While infected with gonorrhea, a woman may have much more menstrual discomfort than she has ordinarily.

Other Sites Of Infection

Gonorrhea can also affect the eyes. If it accidentally spreads to the conjunctiva, it can develop into a serious infection and lead to blindness in the affected eye. This doesn't happen often, but when it does, the blindness may be irreversible. *Early treatment in such cases is urgent.* This problem has been known for over a hundred years, mostly because the one most likely to be stricken in this manner is the infant born to a mother with gonorrhea.

A sore throat can also be due to gonorrhea. Anyone engaging in fellatio (oral sex) who is in contact with an infected penis can develop a gonococcal throat infection. Though this can be a potentially serious infection, complications from it don't usually occur and it is rarely communicable.

Diagnosing Gonorrhea

Only a man with a full-blown case of the disease will, a few days after the infection, show external symptoms that are so obvious that a clinician can diagnose it at once without the help of a laboratory. In some men and in most women there may be only some uncharacteristic, outward evidence—making a laboratory test necessary. At the present time, there are two methods of testing for gonorrhea in common use. These are the "smear" and the "culture." Other methods are in experimental stages.

The smear technique of diagnosis is used with men but rarely with women. A small amount of fluid, or discharge, swabbed from the interior of the penis tip, is called a smear if it's put on a glass slide, dried, and examined in a laboratory. When stained with what is known as a Gram Stain, or with other similar coloring agents, the technician can see the gonococci under a microscope. Appropriately enough, they always appear like lovebirds, two together hiding inside a cell. Side by side, the two resemble a coffee bean.

This method of diagnosis doesn't take very long. Of course, it takes time for the smear to get to the laboratory and for the technician to get to your diagnosis, and then send the information back to the clinic, or to your doctor, and on to you.

The culture method of diagnosis is the preferred method for women. In the female, there are so many bacteria in the vagina that examining a smear on a slide could prove confusing. In a culture, a trifle of discharge is removed from inside the tip of the womb with a swab. Instead of being put on a slide, it's placed in a culture medium that filters out most other bacteria and suppresses them so that only the gonococcus and closely-related germs can grow—which they do, like chicken eggs in an incubator. They multiply to such an extent, in large colonies, that a diagnosis can be readily made. Nonetheless, the technician still double-checks to be sure that what has grown are truly gonococci. Sometimes, if a man has little discharge but gonorrhea is suspected, the culture method is used instead of the smear technique.

The culture method is also used to test whether a cure has been achieved after a course of treatment. This applies to both men and women. Using the culture method for test of cure in men is a precautionary procedure because, after treatment, the discharge may be too scant to prepare a slide, yet gonococci may still be found to grow in a culture.

So far, no reliable blood tests for gonorrhea have been developed. Recently, some tests have become available but their usefulness to accurately diagnose this disease is limited. When you hear of a blood test done to determine if an S.T.D. exists, it is usually a test for syphilis or for AIDS.

Curing Gonorrhea

When treated, it doesn't take long for gonorrhea to be cured—usually only a few days. Even if there is partial resistance by the germs to the first treatment, a second go-around with the same, or with different medication will usually take care of the gonococci. However, the bad news is that some more-resistant organisms are cropping up in increasing numbers and they may pose problems in the future. More about this later on.

You don't need many visits to the clinic or the doctor's office to effect a cure for gonorrhea. The first visit may produce a diagnosis; and, if gonorrhea is found to exist, treatment can begin promptly. About a week later, another visit has to be made to be certain that a cure was effected. If one knows definitely that there was exposure to an infection, or if the outward signs are obvious (often the case with men), then treatment is begun during the first visit, even before there is bacteriological confirmation of the diagnosis.

A second visit is then necessary only for what we call "test of cure." Nowadays, between 90 and 95 percent of all cases are cured with the first round of medicine. However, the other 5 to 10 percent require more of the same, or different, medication. The reason we urge everybody to come back for this test of cure is that the 5 to 10 percent may outwardly appear cured even though the gonococci have survived the treatment. In these instances, people can still infect others.

All of this, of course, applies only if there are no complications and if the infection hasn't spread from the genitals to other parts of the body.

The Drugs Used In The Cure

It was all actually simpler in the 1940s when we used sulfa drugs, which were very effective. But the gonococcus quickly built up resistance to these drugs and learned to ignore them. Then it was found that an injection of penicillin had a rapid effect on these cocci. Some 300,000 units of injected penicillin did the trick. Those were the days when it seemed that "gonorrhea was easier to cure than a cold." Unfortunately, the gonococcus proved highly adaptable to this drug, too. Its resistance increased and, as time passed, we found that the gonococcus could take 600,000 units without being harmed. Then the strain grew still more resistant—first to 1.2 million units, then to 2.4 million units. Now, if we use penicillin at all, we have to start with 4.8 million units of injected penicillin. When we give this dosage, we put half into each buttock. It's a great deal even for a sizeable human buttock.

And so a physician may prefer different treatment methods. He or she may elect to give drugs related to penicillin (such as ampicillin), and give them by mouth. Or, he or she may give other oral antibiotics called tetracyclines, in particular, doxycycline. There is also another injectable drug called Spectinomycin which is effective against these organisms.

One of the reasons why some physicians prefer treatment by injection is that some patients, given medication to take on their own, may take only a part of it, not all. Noticing that the superficial symptoms have disappeared, they keep the rest of the medicine or give it to a friend. Since the total amount the doctor prescribed was essential for a complete cure, the disease may continue to lurk unnoticed, but not inactive.

With a micro-organism as capricious as the gonococcus, treatment methods change from time to time. We're fortunate that it's still sensitive to several drugs, because every patient's coccus may not respond to the same medication. If one medication doesn't work, the clinician has to turn to a different method of treatment. There is no absolute method by which the doctor or clinician can determine in advance whether an infection will respond to a certain kind of drug. However, there is a method-of-sorts that attempts to do that. The labs

Here's how it works. Gonococci taken from an infected patient are left to grow in a culture medium, that is, a mixture of several ingredients such as blood and seaweed. The cocci thrive on this. Then, a number of different drugs are added, in different degrees of dilution, and on various parts of the culture plates. One can find out which drug, and in which dilution, succeeded in killing the organisms. This technique is extensively used in medicine in cases of bacterial infections other than gonorrhea.

If sensitivity testing were done before treating a gonorrhea patient, it would delay the beginning of every treatment. Since, in acute cases, patients are in considerable discomfort, often in pain, they need medication as quickly as possible. Also, and this can be confusing, the laboratory experience is not always duplicated in the patients. On occasion, organisms that in a lab test are found to be highly sensitive to a certain drug, may not respond to it during actual treatment—and vice versa.

Once in a while, a treatment doesn't lead to a prompt cure. There are three possible causes for this. One is that the gonococcus may have become indifferent to the medicine given, or the dose prescribed was too small. Another is that the patient may have become reinfected because his or her sex-mate didn't also come in for treatment. And the third reason may be that the patient didn't take all the medication prescribed. Unfortunately, this does happen.

When a treatment doesn't result in a prompt cure, the physician may sometimes prescribe another round of the same drug. You may ask why, if it didn't work, it should be re-peated. Between the first round and the second, the body's self-curing tendency may have advanced a bit and the weakened organisms may now respond to the renewed treat-ment with antibiotics.

When The Gonococci Don't Respond To Treatment

The number of gonococcal strains resisting treatment with penicillin is rapidly increasing in some parts of the world where drugs are freely available for self-treatment. Under such circumstances, people often give themselves or receive insufficient treatment for their infections. Thus, the organisms which are best able to resist this minimal treatment ("survival of the fittest") are the ones that outlive their weaker counterparts. This makes for strains of highly resistant agents, and such gonococci are invading the U.S. and some European countries. However, although clusters of such organisms have been found here and are spreading around the country, there are still no super-gonococci that can resist every one of the antibiotic treatment methods available to us. As such super-germs develop in the future, we have to try to keep a jump ahead of them with our antibiotic armamentarium.

The subject of self-medication, which is not recommended, leads to the next question: what if someone doesn't get any treatment at all for gonorrhea? Well, we know from the time before antibiotics that it is possible for gonorrhea, eventually, to cure itself. In a man, with luck, such an untreated infection can be cured in anywhere from a number of weeks to many months. In women it takes longer—several weeks to a year or more. But no one can predict if it *will* cure itself, how long it will take, and how much damage may be done to various parts of the body before the body succeeds in fighting off the disease. Furthermore, while the infection exists, a sick person can give it to his or her sex partner. So common sense dictates that treatment is essential. This is an instance where it is senseless to let nature take its course, when medication can speed up recovery and prevent the infection from causing permanent damage.

In summary, the best advice on gonorrhea is this: If you've got it, get rid of it—*fast*. Not by giving it to someone else (that doesn't cure anyone), but by proper medical treatment.

CHAPTER EIGHT

Syphilis
The Facts,
Plus Some Fiction

As I said in the last chapter, one might well ask why a book on the *new* sexually transmitted diseases would include such oldies as gonorrhea and syphilis. Not only does the frequency with which these two diseases now occur put a new slant on their significance as medical problems, but, in the case of syphilis particularly, the gravity of this disease is such that everyone interested in the subject of S.T.D.s should be at least minimally informed about its symptoms, course, and treatment.

Syphilis, one of the more serious S.T.D.s, is caused by a coil-shaped micro-organism called the spirochaete (pronounced *spi-ro-keet*). Its scientific name is treponema pallidum. The scary thing about this germ is that it can attack any tissue or organ in the body.

The origin of the word "syphilis" is amusing—though the disease is anything but. In the sixteenth century, an Italian pathologist named Hieronymus Fracastorius wrote a poem that described the plight of a mythical shepherd named Syphilus who was afflicted with this disease as punishment for cursing the gods. The venereal nature of this disease was mentioned in the poem, and thirty-six years later an English surgeon named Thomas Gale actually introduced the word syphilis into the English language.

Speculation about the origin of syphilis provides one of the most fascinating chapters in any medical history book. Much evidence indicates that the disease came from the New World. One theory, known as the "Columbian Theory," claims that the disease was widespread among Indians in the newly discovered Western world, and the crew of Christopher Columbus' ship picked it up in the area that is today known as Haiti. Then, according to this version, it was carried back to Spain at the end of the fifteenth century, providing the first source of European syphilization.

The tale continues: late in 1494, the French besieged Naples. Their army had many mercenaries and after the fall of Naples, syphilis spread throughout Italy. The occupying army had many cases of the disease and soldiers so afflicted were returned to their homelands, which included nearly every country in Europe. In a short time, the disease was known everywhere on that continent. Of course, this theory doesn't explain how syphilis first got its start in America.

Because of its supposed connection with the French army, the Italians dubbed it "The French Disease," a name that caught on and lasted a couple of hundred years, although it's no longer used. However, since the French army picked it up in Naples, Frenchmen called syphilis "le mal de Naples." For their part, the English preferred to call it "the Spanish disease" because of the large number of Spanish mercenaries in the

French army. Historically speaking, everyone was generous about naming it for someone else.

There are other theories as well concerning the origin of this venereal disease. There are historians who insist vehemently that syphilis existed in Europe before Columbus' voyages, and that it was confused with other diseases, possibly with leprosy. The theories of such historians are referred to as the "Pre-Columbian Theories."

Some believe that the infection originated in Central Africa in a much milder form and was introduced into Europe by travelers and traders. But enough of history, except to add that, in addition to the names mentioned above, syphilis does have some modern appellations. In the vernacular, it is sometimes referred to as "bad blood," "syph," or "pox." One proper medical term for syphilis is Lues (pronounced "Louis"). A "luetic" is a person who has the disease.

Recognizing The Symptoms

In men, if the case is typical and an early one, it is usually possible to recognize the outward symptoms for what they are. It's more difficult with women because the symptoms may be concealed internally. In both men and women, if the first lesion is inside the rectum, it can also go unnoticed.

Usually, the first sign of syphilis is a sore that develops in the primary stage. However, speaking linguistically, it's an improper use of the word since this "sore" doesn't hurt. It can appear as early as two weeks after infection or as late as two months after—sometimes even later than that. Most commonly it shows up in four to six weeks. It's called a chancre (pronounced *shan-ker*) and may look like a big pimple or an open sore, but not like a blister, and it will be reddish brown in color. It will be hard in texture and the surface usually resembles a crater. In size it can be tiny, but it can also be as big as a dime. There might be a single chancre or several, and they are, as I said, painless. At this stage of the disease an infected person can easily pass it along to someone coming in contact with the sore.

It's possible, however, to have syphilis without this symptom. In women the chancre can be internal and smaller, perhaps hidden in the folds of the vagina lining where it can't be seen during an examination. And even in men the sore can be so small as to go unnoticed.

The first sore is likely to be—but not necessarily—in the area of the genitals. It can appear just about anywhere that contact with the infection was originally made: finger, tongue, lip, breast, rectum, or anywhere else in or on the body. Incidentally, syphilis *can* be acquired by kissing alone—but the chances of this happening are remote. Whether visible or not, the chancre is highly contagious at this point because it's loaded with spirochaetes.

By no means are all sores in or around the genital region due to syphilis—or for that matter, to a sexually transmitted disease. While the sores may be suspect until proven harmless, there are many other kinds of sores that also favor the genital area.

The fact that a chancre disappears does not mean that a patient is cured—absolutely not. Even without treatment it will disappear while the spirochaetes remain and spread through the body. On the other hand, treated promptly, it will disappear quickly and with it will go the dangers of developing serious consequences, or of infecting others. If untreated, the chancre will heal within a few weeks, leaving no external sign. This is unfortunate because the infected person may think that whatever had ailed him or her has been cured, which is not the case at all. The spirochaetes spread rapidly and within a few weeks they can be just about everywhere in the body busily producing what we call "secondary syphilis."

About the same time that the chancre appears, the lymph nodes in the groin swell and enlarge. This, again, is usually painless and may go unnoticed. From three to six weeks after the first chancre appears, an infected person might develop a rash that can show up anywhere on the body or *all over the body*. Other symptoms may include a sore throat, headaches, a slight fever and, sometimes, a sort of patchy loss of hair.

Of course, any of these symptoms could be unrelated to syphilis, but an experienced clinician can usually tell whether they have any connection with venereal disease. Syphilis can mimic many other diseases, so the layperson shouldn't attempt to draw any conclusions merely on the basis of symptoms.

Secondary Syphilis

After the disappearance of the chancre or chancres, a skin eruption will usually follow—and this can occur anywhere from a few weeks to a few months later. In its most typical form, this skin rash is widespread and also affects the palms of the hands, and sometimes, the foot soles, as well as the mouth and nose. To the layperson, this rash, if mild, may resemble a heat rash, or even measles—although the color is a bit darker and has a brownish rather than a reddish cast. Some experts get their clue from the hue, and from the way the eruption appears to turn lighter or darker as it goes from the center toward the periphery. But even the most experienced physician can sometimes be misled by what his eye tells him, so a laboratory test is essential for an accurate diagnosis.

Many people infected with syphilis don't recall having had either a sore or a rash. We know that some people never do experience any *secondary* symptoms, but that doesn't happen very often. More frequently, people have merely forgotten that they had the rash. In these cases, it either didn't seem noteworthy at the time or was attributed to an allergy. I once had a patient who didn't, at first, remember having a rash. After further contemplation, he recalled having a skin outbreak that he had thought was a mild case of German measles.

There are other symptoms of secondary syphilis. Lymph nodes become swollen all over the body and an infected person may not feel at all well, suffering mild, flu-like symptoms. These could include a slight temperature, chills, a sore throat, and a feeling of tiredness. Treated or untreated, this stage goes away in a week or two. After that, if untreated, the disease has merely gone underground; the next outward signs could take years to show themselves. The disease is not cured and the patient remains infected, though he may no longer be contagious. Syphilis is most communicable during the primary and secondary stages.

During the secondary stage, if adequately treated, the rash will disappear, the lymph nodes will return to normal, and it's over, a thing of the past, even though blood tests may remain positive for as much as a year or longer. A cured patient is not, however, immune from getting another syphilis infection. The disease can be contracted again, with the cycle beginning all over: primary stage, secondary stage, etc.

The Tertiary Stage

As I said, if untreated, the disease goes underground—and the untreated patient may do so, too, before his or her time. Because syphilis can kill.

The spirochaetes can remain unnoticed in the body for years. But unnoticed doesn't mean inactive. During this latent or quiet stage, the large masses of corkscrew germs scatter throughout the body. The infected person is then into the late or tertiary (third) stage. In this country, we estimate that there are approximately a hundred thousand people who have syphilis and are not being treated for it.

In the late stages of syphilis, the spirochaete can produce heart disease, affect the aorta (the largest blood vessel in the body), and produce serious damage in the brain and in the centers for the spinal nerves. Paralysis, insanity, and even death may result. Once the late stage of syphilis is reached, treatment can still be effective—but damage already done to various parts of the body cannot be undone. At this point, we treat the patient to arrest further progress of the disease.

The Communicable Period

Generally, syphilis can be passed along to another person for about a year after infection. However, it's possible for the infectious period to last as long as two years; in some rare cases, even longer. While a patient becomes non-infectious after one to two years, the disease can be passed along indefinitely to a fetus or newborn baby, or through blood transfusions. Strange as it may seem, the worst damage to the body of a syphilitic will occur *after* he or she has ceased to be infectious.

Blindness And Insanity

Syphilis can affect the eyes, but this usually occurs only in the late stages of the disease—after many years of an untreated or insufficiently treated infection. The disease can damage the eye nerve, the iris (and with it, the size of the pupil), and other parts of the eye, making blindness a distinct possibility. Unfortunately, treatment of these eye conditions is difficult; even antibiotics are of limited help. Eye disorders can also occur in congenital syphilis if the embryo is infected while in the womb.

Syphilitic insanity is much more rare than it was before the days of penicillin—but not as rare as we would like it to be. About one in forty people with untreated syphilis will become insane. We spend more than a hundred million dollars a year treating patients with syphilitic psychoses who are in public institutions, and despite progress being made in this area, some of these people remain incurable.

What I've described about damage that occurs in untreated syphilis is what *usually* happens. But for reasons we don't fully understand, some syphilitic patients escape these late impairments. Perhaps some just don't live long enough to reach the late stages; in others, treatment for some unrelated illness can sometimes take care of the spirochaetes.

Diagnosing Syphilis

The appearance of early syphilis—that is, the primary and secondary stages mentioned above—is usually quite characteristic and suggests this disease to the doctor who sees it. That's not enough, however, because the look of the lesions can be deceiving. Therefore, the diagnosis has to be made with the help of a microscope, a procedure known as a "darkfield examination." If one looks into the microscope, the background appears dark, but anything floating around in a drop of special fluid, including bacteria, will light up like dust particles in a beam of sunshine. This technique enables us to detect the corkscrew-like spirochaete in the early stages of syphilis.

Unfortunately, some people who have a sore will raid the medicine cabinet and find creams, ointments, iodine, or old antibiotics with which they "treat" the lesion. In those cases, they may kill the surface germs, if not the ones deeper down, and make their detection under a microscope impossible.

When the disease has reached a later stage, the diagnosis can only be confirmed by means of a blood test. Early in this century, a German bacteriologist, Dr. August von Wassermann, introduced the first blood test for syphilis. While the actual method has changed considerably over the years, we still hear of the "Wassermann Test." There are almost two hundred other names for it—usually the name of the person who modified the test in some way—although many doctors just refer to it as a "serology" test. The different tests we now use are all good, but only two or three of them are in wide use.

The most popular tests are the VDRL Test (the initials stand for Venereal Disease Research Laboratory), the FTA Absorption Test (FTA stands for Fluorescent Treponema Antibodies), and the RPR Test (Rapid Plasma Reagin). Because the decision about which to use rests with the physician or clinic you visit, it's unimportant for you to be more than passingly familiar with the names, if at all.

Currently, most clinics and doctors use either the VDRL or RPR tests because they're easier to perform, cheaper, quicker (in most places), and generally simpler. They have one disadvantage. Once in a while—and I should point out that this is not a rare occurrence—this test may show a positive result for some reason unrelated to syphilis. We call this a "false positive." If there is even the slightest cause to doubt the results, positive tests are then confirmed by FTA tests, which don't have this disadvantage. The principal reason the FTA isn't used routinely is that ordinarily it can't be done locally. Because the test may have to be done in another town, it can take a week or more until the results are back. It's not 100 percent reliable, either, although it comes close.

When someone becomes infected, it will be one to two months before a VDRL test will become positive; a somewhat shorter time for the FTA test. In secondary syphilis they are both always positive, or what we call "reactive."

The RPR test is relatively simple and, as the name says, it's *rapid*. Results can be obtained within hours, from a blood sample. This test is a reliable substitute for the VDRL and is in wide use; but, as with the latter test, there are also occasional false positive results. It's up to the clinician whether or not a test result should be confirmed with the more complicated and time-consuming FTA test.

Meaning Of "False Positive"

As I said, once in a while a VDRL or RPR test will show a "false positive" result and sometimes remain so, for unknown reasons, in a perfectly healthy individual. In these cases, however, the FTA test will be negative.

The presence of another disease can also create a "false positive" result. For instance, some tropical diseases, including malaria, can trigger such a reaction. It also occasionally occurs in heroin users. And, for a short while after acute viral infections, a person could also show such a reaction, although this is relatively rare.

Treatment Of Syphilis

One massive shot (2.4 million units) of a special, long-acting type of penicillin will usually bring the disease under control if the infection was recently acquired. In many cases, this is followed by a second injection a week later. If the infection is older, a third shot is added, about a week after that. This is in great contrast to the days before penicillin when it required a year and a half of unpleasant and often risky weekly injections to control the infection—*maybe*.

These were injections with Ehrlich's "606"—the 606th preparation in his search for a chemical that could be used as the "magic bullet" against syphilis. It was said in those days that the only *certain* cure for the disease was embalming fluid. There were also attempted cures with bismuth and with arsenic—substances that weren't beneficial to the body. Sometimes deafness and other side effects resulted from the treatment, but people were willing to take chances to fight the disease. Sir Alexander Fleming, the discoverer of penicillin, changed all that for us.

When discussing treatment for gonorrhea, I mentioned that bigger and bigger doses of antibiotics are needed because the gonococcus is so adaptable and stubborn. Fortunately, this does not apply to the spirochaetes causing syphilis. They have not changed. As a matter of fact, we now need bigger doses of penicillin to cure gonorrhea than to treat early syphilis.

Once in a while there are reports of some isolated cases of super-spirochaetes that resist treatment; but usually, if a chancre doesn't respond to treatment with penicillin, the sore was probably not syphilitic but chancroid.

If someone is known to be allergic to penicillin, it's necessary for that person to swallow a large number of capsules containing another antibiotic. These are taken over a period of from two to four weeks, and not every stomach can take it. This is one reason why it's undesirable to take penicillin for minor ailments—it's a drug that should not be used unless there's very good reason to do so. The repeated use of penicillin can make some people allergic ("sensitive") to it—in which case it won't be available to them when an illness or disease really requires it.

The longer a person has a syphilitic infection before getting treatment, the longer it will take for his or her blood tests to return to normal. In a recent infection, treated early, it still takes between six months and a year. If the infection existed for a year or two before treatment, it may take several years before the blood is again negative or "non-reactive." But if the infection is of even longer duration, it may never again become "non-reactive." Even though cured, such a person's blood test can remain positive for life. The FTA test, once positive, usually remains so for life, even if the person is cured. This test, therefore, is of no use to determine whether someone has been adequately treated.

Contagiousness

Once the course of treatment for syphilis is completed, a person is no longer contagious, regardless of whether the blood test shows a positive reaction. When the doctor says that the non-contagious stage has been reached, sexual relations are permissible despite the fact that a test might remain reactive.

Non-Venereal Syphilis

The term "non-venereal syphilis" refers to this disease when it's acquired without intimate sexual contact. This can occur in a lab worker or nurse who accidentally injures herself or himself with a needle that's been used on a syphilitic patient. This is a rare occurrence.

Another type of non-venereal syphilis exists in some hot countries with rather primitive hygienic standards. Such infections are known by other names, depending upon the country where the disease occurs. One of these names is "Bejel." The germ causing this disease is not distinguishable from the spirochaete causing syphilis, but the characteristics of the ailment are different. While it affects many parts of the body other than the sex organs, the late consequences to organs are less serious; the heart and brain are almost never affected. And the disease is more common in children. Yaws, another infection that used to be common in hot countries with low sanitary standards, belongs in the same category. Some people believe that these diseases are the "Stone Age" syphilis from which present-day syphilis may have evolved.

Control Of Syphilis

There was a time, perhaps twenty years ago, when we thought that with the help of penicillin, syphilis could be wiped out and go the route of many other communicable diseases which are a thing of the past—diseases such as polio, tetanus, smallpox, and so on. But that goal has not been achieved. In fact, syphilis is still a widely prevalent health threat. Many have lost the fear of syphilis; since there appears to be great confidence that treatment is available to cure it, some people have become casual about this disease. There are too many indifferent transmitters.

In the United States and its territories, the rate of reported cases per hundred thousand people has declined slightly in recent years. It is currently highest in Los Angeles. The next nine cities, in descending order of frequency of occurrence, are New York, Chicago, Houston, Philadelphia, San Francisco, Miami, Washington, D.C., Baltimore, and Atlanta.

CHAPTER NINE

Three Rare
Venereal Diseases

We usually use the older, more limiting term, "venereal disease," when categorizing three other infectious diseases acquired through sexual contact. These are chancroid, granuloma inguinale, and lympho-granuloma venereum, often referred to as LGV.

All three of these diseases can be quite troublesome and difficult to diagnose and treat; physicians may be unfamiliar with them because they are seen so rarely. However, a physician specializing in this field or a clinician in a regional V.D. clinic can almost always diagnose and treat all three of the diseases.

Anyone who travels to parts of the world with low hygienic standards and is sexually active should be warned that these diseases are common in such places. For example, in the early '70s the incidence of chancroid among troops in Southeast Asia was quite high, and returning military personnel re-introduced it into parts of this country where it didn't previously exist. Let's take the three diseases one at a time.

Chancroid

Chancroid originally got its name because of its similarity in appearance to the chancre of syphilis. However, a syphilitic lesion is harder in consistency, not usually painful, and, upon a darkfield microscopic examination, yields findings of spirochaetes, which chancroid does not.

Chancroid is found more frequently in men than women—three times more often, in fact. In men, the disease may show itself in single or multiple lesions on the external genitals or the anus. Women can be asymptomatic or experience only a mild vaginitis. If lesions do occur, they will generally be on the labia, clitoris, anus or cervix, and such lesions will be tender. However, since similar lesions may also occur in syphilis, diagnosis first requires a microscopic examination of a sample from the lesion in order to eliminate the possible presence of spirochaetes; then a special staining procedure is done. This staining procedure is a complicated one that can usually be done only in special V.D. centers.

The treatment of chancroid takes patience and time—usually ten to fourteen days, but sometimes longer. The organisms that cause this disease are becoming increasingly resistant to the tetracyclines, which are ordinarily used to treat it. Where there is a resistant strain, the disease can be treated with combinations of other antibiotics that are quite effective. One such antibiotic is erythromycin. Sometimes, other drugs have to be administered intramuscularly several times a day for a week before a cure is effected.

Granuloma Inguinale

Granuloma inguinale is caused by a small bacillus and is a disease that's fairly common in countries of low sanitary standards. In the United States, the number of reported cases is very small—almost nil in the northern part of the country.

This disease has a relatively long incubation period—from eight to twelve weeks. At first it produces little nodules under the skin, usually around the genitals. In time, the covering skin erodes and beefy-red lesions appear, usually painless. Since these can easily be mistaken for syphilitic lesions, darkfield examinations are necessary to ascertain that no spirochaetes are present.

In granuloma inguinale, the picture in the microscope shows cells characteristic of the disease. They are known as "Donovan bodies." If the disease is allowed to progress, it can lead to strictures (narrowing of the urethra or the anal canal) and large scar formations which remain even after the disease is treated and cured. This infection, too, responds to prolonged courses of antibiotics.

Lympho-Granuloma Venereum (LGV)

This disease is caused by an organism that belongs to the chlamydia group and is closely related to the chlamydia that causes non-gonococcal urethritis. (See Chapter 4.) However, the manifestations of the disease are very difficult from non-gonococcal urethritis. At first, LGV produces painless little ulcers usually located, in women, on the vaginal wall or the cervix. In men, the ulcers might appear on the skin of the genitals or anus. These ulcers are rarely diagnosed for what they are. Since the ulcers are painless and are, in women, inside the body and therefore unnoticed, the disease doesn't usually prompt a visit to the doctor for a diagnosis.

As the disease progresses, the ulcers enlarge, fistulas are formed, and often the rectum becomes involved, producing strictures, pain and constipation. It is then that medical care is frequently sought.

Treating this disease calls for patience—it takes time. However, once properly diagnosed, it does respond to some antibiotics, including tetracyclines, that require a minimum of two to three weeks of treatment before a cure is achieved.

Although LGV occurs only rarely in this country, its presence in Southeast Asia makes it a possibility here. A diagnostician must take this into account.

CHAPTER TEN

Other Sexually Transmissible Diseases

Practically every communicable disease can be transmitted through the close contact of sexual relations. This would include various forms of the streptococcal and meningo-coccal infections, the flu, and even colds, if you stretch the point. These illnesses, however, are customarily treated as though they were *not* sexually transmitted. More properly, they should be spoken of as sexually *transmissible* diseases, indicating that they *could* be passed along by sexual contact.

Other sexually transmissible diseases are trichomoniasis and candidiasis (discussed in Chapter 5, which deals with various types of vaginitis), venereal warts caused by the human papilloma virus, crab lice, and scabies (Chapter 15, *Sexually Transmitted Skin Conditions*), and those infections caused by intestinal microorganisms that, during anal intercourse, can be transferred out of their conventional locale and environment. (These infections are covered in Chapter 17, *S.T.D.s in the Gay Community*.) Other sexually transmissible diseases, described below, include infections with the cytomegalovirus, the Epstein-Barr virus, mycoplasma and Group B streptococcal infections, as well as hepatitis B.

The Cytomegalovirus (CMV)

Infections with CMV are common; in fact, almost half of all people have, or have had, this infection. Most CMV infections produce no symptoms at all or, at most, a few days of general malaise. On the other hand, severe cases of cytomegalovirus have been known to cause permanent body damage, even death.

CMV is a member of the herpes virus family, but the signs of this infection are very different from those seen after a herpes simplex infection. It shares with the herpes virus one particular characteristic: once an infection is acquired, it can lie dormant, and then flare up during periods of reduced immunity.

When a recently acquired CMV infection does produce symptoms, they may merely be those associated with an elevated temperature. Apart from the fever, this disease can have a variety of manifestations: fatigue, joint and muscle pains, swollen lymph nodes, and a sense of dragging oneself around. The severity of the illness can vary greatly from no symptoms at all to all of those listed above.

The CMV doesn't survive outside the body—it's transmitted directly from person to person. Because the virus is present in both saliva and sperm (where it can live for a long time), both kissing and sexual intercourse are modes of transmission, which is why the disease is usually included in any list of

S.T.D.s. In fact, in 5 to 10 percent of young, healthy adults, CMV can be found on cultures from saliva or from the cervix. For this reason, sexual contact is considered the principal mode of transmission in young adults, although not the only one. CMV can also be contracted through blood transfusions, and the newborn can acquire the infection from its mother either directly (while in the womb or during delivery) or through milk in breast feeding.

Suspicion of a CMV infection can be verified through lab tests by taking cultures on samples of urine, blood, or from the throat. The CMV can be cultured from the blood only during the acute phase of the illness while, in urine or saliva, CMV can be very persistent and found even years after the primary infection took place.

Because it's an organism that's very difficult to grow, CMV cultures can often be negative despite the presence of the virus. For this reason, many clinicians prefer an alternate method of testing—that is, blood examinations (serological complement fixation tests). Such testing, however, takes time because one has to see if there is a difference in antibodies against CMV over the course of two to three weeks. At least two specimens have to be compared, and they have to be taken ten to fourteen days apart.

Unfortunately, there is no treatment for CMV. All one can do is control the symptoms, if there are any. Nonetheless, it's of value to establish a diagnosis in order to rule out the presence of a treatable infection, and to clarify symptoms that might otherwise be unexplained. There has been extensive investigation of vaccines that might prevent this infection but, at this time, none is ready for practical use. Research, however, is still going on and perhaps some breakthrough may be in the offing.

Mycoplasmas

Even among micro-organisms, the mycoplasmas are small. They come in many species and strains, some of which cause venereal disease and abortions in animals; while others are capable of causing pneumonia in humans, an infection that used to be known as "atypical pneumonia." Still others in this group can cause non-gonococcal urethritis, prostatitis and salpingitis. Infection with one subspecies called ureaplasma urealyticum is common in the human genital tract, although it often seems to have no adverse effect on the body.

In some animal species, particularly cattle and horses, the mycoplasmas can cause infertility. There is hot debate going on in the medical community as to whether or not they could occasionally cause sterility in humans.

These micro-organisms respond to treatment with tetracyclines and erythromycin. Since their role in infertility is uncertain, some physicians play it safe and, in cases of unexplained difficulty in conceiving, treat for the disease even if no symptoms are evident.

"Infectious Mononucleosis"

What used to be called "infectious mononucleosis" is usually a benign disease caused by the Epstein-Barr virus, a member of the herpes group of viruses.

Although not too much is known about the exact method of transmission, it's usually included among the sexually transmitted diseases because of its high prevalence in the age group in which S.T.D.s peak, and because the virus is present in saliva—the reason the infection is also known as "the kissing disease."

Infections with the Epstein-Barr virus, often referred to as "Mono," are usually rather mild but they can also be quite troublesome and incapacitating, with irregular fever, sore throat, swollen lymph nodes, and an enlarged spleen. Because, if symptomatic, the illness can last for many weeks, even months, it frequently leaves a person quite debilitated.

Since the symptoms are often vague and vary from individual to individual, a diagnosis would be difficult to make on clinical grounds alone, were it not for the fact that there are some characteristic changes in the blood during this illness. But even after a diagnosis has been made, there is no specific treatment other than rest and possibly aspirin or other medication to alleviate the symptoms.

Group B Streptococcus

This is an organism that can be transmitted in many ways, including kissing and sexual intercourse. Although it can cause a variety of symptoms, the most common being a sore throat, it doesn't usually produce severe illness in an adult.

However, it's a significant organism among the S.T.D.s because it can infect an embryo or newborn infant, in whom it can cause serious consequences. Fortunately, this occurs rarely. Infections of the cervix with Group B streptococci are common—as many as twenty to thirty percent of all young adult women carry the organism—but only a few clinics routinely test for it in pregnant women because, even if the organism is found, treatment is not entirely without risk.

Hepatitis

Hepatitis is an infection that is now included among S.T.D.s even though there are many ways, other than sexual contact, that one can acquire it.

Later on, in Chapter 17 *(S.T.D.s in the Gay Community),* I will go into more detail about hepatitis and will discuss the special risk of this infection in the homosexual male population. In this section, I will provide only some general comments about the disease.

Infections with any of the three types of hepatitis, called A, B, and non-A, non-B, may carry no noticeable symptoms. When there are signs of the disease, they can occur in all degrees of severity, depending upon individual susceptibility and on how heavy the exposure to the virus has been.

Most such illnesses are mild. One of the more evident signs is a yellow discoloration of the white of the eye and of the fingernails; and, sometimes, there is also a yellowing of the skin. This is known as jaundice—the French word for yellow is *jaune.* However, such yellowing occurs in only ten percent of all hepatitis cases.

An infection with one of the hepatitis viruses confers lifelong immunity on the person who's had it—you can't be reinfected with the same viral strain. But there is no cross-immunity among the three types of hepatitis—having hepatitis A will not provide immunity against hepatitis B.

Hepatitis A is usually contracted through food—when food is uncooked (as in raw seafood); undercooked; or—after cooling—touched by unclean human hands. Hepatitis B, formerly known as serum hepatitis (also as homologous serum jaundice) is *not* foodborne. The virus is present in blood, saliva, and sperm, so it can be transmitted sexually or through shared needles among drug users. Because this virus can survive outside of the body, it can also be transmitted by other types of exposure, usually unknown.

The third type of hepatitis, non-A, non-B, is an infection about which we know relatively little. The source is obvious when the infection takes place after a blood transfusion but we know there must be other means of transmission as well, although we're not certain what they are. Although there are blood tests which can tell us whether a person has, or has had, hepatitis A or B, no such test exists at this time for the third type.

Preventing Hepatitis

Immune-serum Globulin, better known as gamma globulin, is given to prevent hepatitis, but this serum protects one only against hepatitis A. There is a special type of gamma globulin that can prevent type B but it is in short supply, is expensive, and is only of limited duration in effectiveness. For these reasons, it's used only for definite cases of recent, massive exposure, as when someone is accidentally pricked with a needle known to have been contaminated.

A hepatitis B vaccine (Heptavax-B) has been licensed for use in this country. It's given in three intramuscular injections over a six-month period; but such vaccines are not intended for the general population, only for selected groups at high risk of acquiring hepatitis B. This would include certain categories of health care workers as well as persons who have numerous sex partners.

The duration of effectiveness of this vaccine is still unknown but it *appears* that protection is provided for at least five years. After that period, a booster may become necessary if immunity is to be maintained. Side effects from this vaccine have been mild and of short duration.

CHAPTER ELEVEN

S.T.D.s in Pregnancy
Protecting the Unborn

Both gonorrhea and syphilis can have adverse effects on the embryo, as well as on the pregnant woman herself. Infections with chlamydia and herpes may not seriously affect the mother-to-be beyond the effects they would have on a non-pregnant woman, but they can present a danger to the newborn if it is infected before or during birth. Cytomegalovirus, a virus in the herpes family, is widespread nowadays and may occasionally, if infrequently, affect a newborn infant. When this virus is present, there is no preventive measure that can be taken to avoid damage to the newborn. Monilia (candida) discussed on page 53, is an organism commonly present in the vagina. It thrives during pregnancy but its presence is more a nuisance than a menace.

Finally, any organism that can cause an infection, such as the streptococcus, is capable of harming the embryo or the newborn infant, although the probability is remote. Statistically speaking, if one were to treat every pregnant woman for every micro-organism that might be found in her body, the treatment itself would carry as much risk as the infection. Physicians, therefore, have to make decisions on an individual basis, case by case, as to whether or not treatment is indicated.

Chlamydial Infections In Pregnancy

Chlamydial infections (discussed in detail in Chapter 4) in pregnant women are associated with higher rates of premature births and of stillbirths. This is not to say that such an infection will *always* result in either of these—it's just that they happen, statistically speaking, with greater frequency than in the population at large.

One potentially dangerous consequence of a chlamydial infection during pregnancy is that the infant may become infected during birth. This could lead to conjunctivitis and to a low-grade pneumonia. Fortunately, both of these illnesses respond to antibiotics.

If a man is suffering from an S.T.D., his sperm will not affect the embryo as far as infections are concerned. However, the man can, and probably will infect the mother; and her illness, in turn, can adversely affect the pregnancy.

Effect Of S.T.D.s On Fertility

In both women and men, the narrow ducts through which the egg or sperm travels may get blocked by inflammation and make passage impossible. Sometimes such damage is reversible with treatment; other times it isn't. No one should assume that because of gonorrhea or a chlamydial infection pregnancy is impossible. In some prenatal clinics as many as 8 percent of the pregnant women have been found to be infected with gonorrhea, and the percentage is even higher for chlamydia.

Tubal Pregnancies

It is possible for an existing, or even past infection, to cause a pregnancy in the Fallopian tubes because, when the tubes are partially blocked either by inflammation or scar tissue, the fertilized egg may not reach the uterus. If it remains in the tube, where the walls are too thin to support a growing egg, the wall will eventually break, requiring an emergency operation to remove both the tube and the egg. Fortunately, there is a spare tube, and if it's in good shape it remains available to transport an egg from the ovary to the uterus on future occasions.

Preventing Eye Infections And Blindness

Gonococcal eye infection in the newborn used to be one of the most common causes of blindness. More than a hundred and fifty years ago an obstetrician named Karl Credé introduced a method of putting a drop of silver nitrate in each eye of every baby born, to kill any harmful micro-organism that might be present. This procedure has greatly reduced the incidence of infant blindness due to this cause, and it's still used today. In some states the law requires the routine instillation of these drops, whether or not the mother has an infection. Even with the introduction of antibiotics, this preventive method hasn't changed much, although some physicians prefer antibiotics over silver nitrate.

Syphilis, Fertility, And The Fetus

Syphilis affects fertility differently. Conception can take place in an infected person but the embryo can die at any stage of development. Among those who do survive there may be congenital syphilis, with defects at birth, or disabilities that don't become evident until later in life.

Syphilis can damage nearly every organ of the unborn. When symptoms are seen, they usually affect the skin, the lining of the nose and mouth, and the bones; and such infants are likely to have big bellies and anemia. Or, the embryo might be stillborn, or grossly malformed. Occasionally, it can be born apparently normal but develop symptoms of syphilis early or later in life. A blood test at birth can help determine whether an infant has become infected.

When congenital syphilis shows up later in life, the symptoms can range from mild to serious—the most serious ones being blindness or other diseases of the eyes, deafness, disorders of the bones and skin, or a peculiar development of the teeth, which have an abnormal shape or are "notched."

The phrase "congenital syphilis" does not mean the disease has been "inherited" in the usual sense of the word—it is not transmitted through the genes. It can, however, be acquired while in the womb. Strangely, congenital syphilis is not infectious—someone who has it cannot transmit it through sexual contact.

Testing For S.T.D.s During Pregnancy

When pregnancy is established, the same test is done as before marriage—a blood test to determine if the woman has syphilis. In most states the law requires these tests. Depending on a woman's sexual history and the possibility of exposure, blood tests for HIV (infection with the AIDS virus) may be added.

In some population groups and certain geographic areas where the likelihood of finding gonorrhea is high, tests for that disease are also carried out routinely. Some physicians also add other tests and examinations—for chlamydia, for herpes, and for streptococci. These are not routinely done; doctors decide what to look for on an individual basis.

Treatment Of S.T.D.s During Pregnancy

Taking medicines while pregnant is, generally speaking, discouraged. However, the risk to the embryo or newborn when certain S.T.D.s are present may be sufficiently serious to warrant medical treatment of the infection. Penicillin as a drug is quite safe for use during pregnancy, unless an individual is allergic to it. Tetracyclines, however, should not be given since they are capable of discoloring teeth of the child and can sometimes affect the bones as well. There is another group of drugs, known as the erythromycins, that can be used during pregnancy if a woman is infected with gonorrhea or syphilis and is allergic to penicillin.

An infection with the AIDS virus (HIV), even when a woman has no symptoms of the disease and appears to be perfectly healthy, presents a serious menace to the embryo or newborn child. The woman may transmit the virus and, at any time—even years later—the child may develop the symptoms of the Acquired Immunodeficiency Syndrome with all its consequences. Yet the mother, though a carrier of the virus, may remain seemingly healthy. For this reason, it is advisable to avoid pregnancy if blood tests are confirmed to be positive for an HIV infection.

CHAPTER TWELVE

Douching

Should You or Shouldn't You?

Vaginal douches have been used for thousands of years for both cleansing purposes and for contraception. There is evidence that Egyptian women used douches some 3500 years ago in order to prevent pregnancy. The rich Greek and Roman women had "douche maidens" among their slaves, who were stationed next to the marital bedroom so that they could administer douches to their mistresses immediately after intercourse, on the assumption that the procedure could prevent a pregnancy.

This commonly held belief about the contraceptive value of douching has never been substantiated. The truth is that they are pretty useless for that purpose. Live sperm cells have been found in the human Fallopian tubes less than two minutes after ejaculation, which means that it's virtually impossible to douche early enough after intercourse to have it serve as a useful contraceptive method.

Others believe that a venereal infection can be prevented by a douche carried out promptly after intercourse. Sometimes it does work, but it's a most unreliable technique. The European bidet was never effective for this purpose, either.

A third purpose ascribed to douching is that it serves as a general cleansing device in personal hygiene. However, if you have no particular problem, there's really no need for it.

Unnecessary Douching

There was a time earlier in this century when we knew less about micro-organisms and it was considered good practice for everyone to be regularly purged, enemaed, douched, gargled, and scrubbed in order to be rid of all those nasty little bacteria. Now we know that this can be overdone. The body has some very effective defenses against many germs; other micro-organisms are useful and shouldn't be destroyed at all. This applies particularly to the healthy vagina or rectum. Unnecessary douching can provoke trouble. This is not to say, of course, that there aren't justified indications for douching.

Vaginal Odors

Bacteria in the vagina which produce unattractive odors can sometimes be treated by douching. But different species of micro-organisms respond to different chemical ingredients, so if you have such a problem, you really should ask a physician's advice. You should get a medical opinion for another reason, too. Some odor-producing organisms are better treated by taking medicine orally, rather than by douching.

Indications For Douching

If it's for the purpose of preventing an S.T.D., douching must take place immediately after intercourse. However, as I said above, it's really not dependable for this purpose. If you use a douche for other reasons, once or twice a week should be the limit, unless a physician has told you otherwise.

Should you douche, use only *low* water pressure. That means the water bag should be no higher than a foot above the nozzle, which will result in a gentle rinsing rather than the action of a water cannon. Greater pressure can force infected material into the womb and beyond it, into the tubes, triggering distressing inflammatory diseases of the pelvis. If you use a bulb type of douche, the pressure exerted on the bulb should also be moderate.

Just before, during, and after the menses, douching should be particularly gentle, with minimal water pressure. The reason for this is that the cervical canal, the passageway leading to the womb and beyond, is open and material from the vagina can be swept up into areas where it has no right to be. This starts infections and, sometimes, P.I.D.

If you've concluded that I am not in favor of routine douching, you're right.

What To Use In A Douche

Through the centuries, a great variety of substances have been added to douches: blossoms, soap, rose extracts, pepper, zinc sulfate, and even wine. Some years back a rumor circulated in the south that the soft drink 7-Up could prevent both pregnancy and infection; the beverage was widely used for that purpose until experience showed up the myth for what it was.

If you do use a douche for some special reason, one table-spoon of ordinary household vinegar in a quart of warm water is safe and as good as most special preparations you can buy in the store. There are, of course, preparations you can buy for this purpose. If your doctor has told you to use one, or has given you a prescription for one, then there's a special reason for it. Sometimes a specific chemical will be prescribed to combat a medical condition that's been diagnosed. Obviously, in such instances, you'll want to use that douche.

The FDA has finally concerned itself with douches as over-the-counter products available to the public. A panel was man-dated to determine the effectiveness, safety, and labelling of such products. When it was found that douches are only vague-ly defined on their packages, the FDA created its own defini-tion. They defined the vaginal douche as a liquid preparation used to "irrigate the vagina over an indeterminate period of time for a variety of purposes." Listed among those purposes were these: cleansing, soothing and refreshing effects, deodorizing, relieving irritations, reducing infective or-ganisms, and altering the pH of the vagina in order to encour-age the growth of normal vaginal flora.

Generally speaking, however, it's better to leave the va-gina alone. If you do douche, don't overdo it. Keep the pres-sure low, and remember that the more you dilute your prepa-ration, the better off you'll probably be.

CHAPTER THIRTEEN

Ailments Linked
to S.T.D.s

As I mentioned earlier in the chapters dealing with these diseases, syphilis can attack just about every organ in the body; and the gonococci and chlamydia, which are a bit more choosey, have their own favorite targets outside the genital area. Their predilection is for the joints and the liver—more precisely, the lining that covers the liver. Such an attack by the gonococci or the chlamydia can produce an ailment that mimics the symptoms one would find in a gallbladder attack. However, pain in the upper right side of the belly of a young, sexually active person is more likely due to an S.T.D. than to gallbladder disease. When an S.T.D. spreads to this area, it's called "peri-hepatitis."

Arthritis And S.T.D.s

While most cases of arthritis are unconnected to sexually transmitted diseases, gonorrhea, chlamydial infections, and syphilis can all produce certain types of arthritis. When a young person develops arthritis due to an S.T.D., it is often difficult to distinguish it from arthritis due to other causes; in fact, it requires considerable skill and experience to tell one from the other. In someone in the late teens, for example, a joint affliction due to rheumatic fever may, when the ailment is new, appear very similar to one caused by gonorrhea. It's true that the gonococcus has its favorite joints; but the micro-organism can be very tricky: occasionally, it will attack *any* joint. I've seen a gonococcal arthritis in the sacroiliac joint of a 44-year-old man. Admittedly, this is most uncommon, but a physician has to keep in mind even the rare possibilities.

Arthritis connected to a venereal disease is seen more often in women than in men. The reason for this is, as I've said elsewhere, that men usually come for treatment of an S.T.D. earlier than women, principally because they suffer more discomfort. Women, often unaware of their infection, may remain untreated and develop complications, one of which can be a painful and sometimes destructive form of arthritis.

Because gonorrhea is so common today, gonococcal joint trouble is also not uncommon. Arthritis caused by syphilis, on the other hand, is something we hardly ever see nowadays. The reason is that such arthritis occurs in syphilitics in the *late* stages of the disease, and more people with syphilis are achieving an early cure. When we find arthritis connected to gonorrhea, we usually see it within weeks after the original infection began.

Reiter's Syndrome

Another form of arthritis is associated with conjunctivitis and urethritis. When these three symptoms occur together, it's known as Reiter's Syndrome, named after the man who first described the ailment. Only lately have we begun to link this syndrome with chlamydiae as the causal agent, and that is still a tentative conclusion.

This type of arthritis most often affects the joints of the legs. It takes only a few weeks after the infection sets in for the symptoms to show up. Such symptoms can range from very mild to severely disabling and, although they tend to disappear in weeks, or even days, they often come back. Such recurrences are common—which is not true of gonococcal arthritis.

Spreading Of Skin Infections

Later on, in the chapter on *Sexually Transmitted Skin Conditions* (pp. 125-131) I will go into some detail on the subject of S.T.D.s which affect the skin. And, in the chapter on *Herpes* (pp. 23-35) I talked about the many areas on the body where this ailment can appear. One of the most serious complications of herpes occurs when the virus affects the brain and produces a form of encephalitis. This is so rare, however, that herpes sufferers (who have enough to worry about) shouldn't lose any sleep over the possibility. True, such a complication is possible. But it's a thousand times more likely that one can be in a serious car accident—yet most of us don't lose much sleep worrying about *that* possibility.

Pain After Intercourse—In Men

Some men experience pain after intercourse. This may be experienced as mild discomfort, as itching, as burning, or as an uncomfortable and frequent urge to urinate; or it can be a severe pain. There are several possible causes for such symptoms.

If the pain is at the very tip of the penis, it is called *meatitis* because the entrance to the male urethra is the *meatus*. We find this type of pain more frequently in non-circumcised men whose foreskin is difficult to retract and who may have problems with hygiene.

But *meatitis* also occurs in the circumcised male. Vaginal infections of the sex partner must then be considered as a possible cause; the woman should be examined and treated if an infection is found.

There are other possible causes for such discomfort or pain after intercourse. One of these is known as a urethral stricture, a narrowing of the urethra due to instrumentation (during an examination) or to a previous infection. Occasionally, a small calculus (a tiny kidney stone) on its way out can injure the urethra or even lodge there temporarily.

But the most common cause of pain after intercourse is an inflammation of the prostate that can require repeated prostatic massage and hot baths several times a day. Sometimes, if bacterial prostatitis is suspected, antibiotics are prescribed. Cystitis after sexual activity is common in women but hardly ever occurs in men. Cystitis is discussed in Chapter 14 (pp. 119-123).

AIDS is a whole different story inasmuch as it can produce a great variety of infections that persons not afflicted by AIDS would fight off. These complications are described in Chapter 18, *AIDS*.

CHAPTER FOURTEEN

Conditions Confused with the Venereal Diseases

There are a number of symptoms in both men and women that can make one suspect the possibility of a venereal disease—provided, of course, that there's been some questionable sexual contact. Some of these symptoms are very similar to the ones that *do* indicate an S.T.D., though no such disease may be present. Professional diagnosis is essential if an accurate picture is to be had on what's going on.

Discharges From The Penis

A man may experience an urgency to urinate, along with some burning sensation and possibly a slight discharge. While such conditions may well be due to an

S.T.D., they can also be linked to cystitis (an inflammation of the bladder), or to a prostatic inflammation.

A discharge from the penis, by itself, by no means proves that an S.T.D. is present. However, among young people (teens and those in their twenties), particularly if the person reports a dubious sexual contact, such a discharge is usually indicative of one of the more common S.T.D.s. Appropriate tests will usually provide a correct diagnosis, and treatment can then be initiated.

Vaginal Discharges

Vaginal discharges are a very common complaint among women of all ages but the presence of such a discharge, which can range from a small amount to a substantial one, can have a number of explanations, some of which are not related to any S.T.D. Where there is a small vaginal discharge unaccompanied by an itch or irritation, it is usually clear or whitish in color and may indicate no abnormality at all. At the other extreme, a discharge can be substantial, annoying, or even distressing, and could be due to an inflammation of the vagina or an organ higher up in the genital tract. Even then it need not necessarily be due to a sexually transmitted disease.

About halfway between two periods, a discharge may appear that is slightly blood-tinged. This is connected with ovulation and is neither abnormal nor anything to be concerned about.

A vaginal discharge, even if it's accompanied by an odor, is not a disease by itself—it's a symptom of something that needs exploration. Sometimes the cause can be as simple and innocuous as tight-fitting, non-absorbent underwear or some harmless, if misplaced, intestinal parasite; or even a foreign body deep in the vagina, such as a small, detached piece of a menstrual tampon.

Chemical vaginitis, discussed earlier in the chapter on *Douching* (pp. 111-114) is due to contact of the vaginal mucosa with inappropriate chemical compounds. This is an ailment that's not transmitted sexually although it sometimes triggers concern about the possibility of a venereal disease.

Cystitis In Women

Cystitis, characterized by frequency of urination and burning or other bladder problems, occurs much more frequently in women than in men. The great majority of women whose complaints suggest bladder infections do not have a sexually transmitted disease. In young, sexually active men, however, frequency of urination along with a burning sensation are usually telltale signs of such an infection.

Frequency of urination in women can be accompanied by distressing pain as the bladder is emptied, by low back aches, and by some blood in the urine. Most commonly this is due to a bladder infection while, in men, the inflammation is more often limited to the urethra, the exit-duct from the bladder. When such symptoms occur in a woman, they call for bacteriological exploration in order to provide the most effective treatment. Different bacteria respond to different drugs, so knowing which one is the culprit tells the physician what to prescribe.

There is a condition known as "honeymoon cystitis," usually caused by mechanical irritation of the short, female urethra. This can be rather painful. Again, proper diagnosis is necessary so that treatment (often no more than warm baths and temporary sexual abstinence) can be initiated.

Skin Conditions Confused With S.T.D.s

A skin eruption in the genital area is by no means necessarily a sign of a sexually transmitted disease. Practically every skin disorder could, by chance, make its appearance in that part of the body. For example, psoriasis, a common skin disorder but certainly not an S.T.D., can appear on the skin of the penis. Another skin condition unrelated to S.T.D.s is "Jean" folliculitis, an inflammation and often an infection of the hair follicles due to wearing jeans that are too tight—it's the body's way of letting you know that it wasn't meant to be encased in such constricting garments. When very tight garments are worn, friction, perspiration, and moisture in this area of the body contribute to the growth of fungal and other micro-organisms. "Jock itch," another common disorder, is not a very scientific name but it's a descriptive one and a good example of what I'm talking about.

Nor is the genital region spared from other dermatological conditions, unrelated to S.T.D.s. Even poison ivy of the penis occurs; and women who happen to sit in a poison ivy patch—sometimes on nude beaches—can develop this annoying contact dermatitis on their genital area.

Allergies that create a reddening and itching of the skin can be due to hypersensitivity to deodorants, cosmetics, and contraceptive creams, as well as to garments made of synthetic materials. For people who have this problem, wearing cotton underwear is a good idea.

Both men and women may sometimes notice wounds and little ulcers in the genital area and, if there's been a questionable sexual contact, an S.T.D. might be suspected. However, such symptoms can, at times, be of a traumatic nature—that is, due to abrasions or bite wounds. Because such lesions can easily become infected with common micro-organisms, proper diagnosis is necessary. If found to be of a traumatic nature, keeping the area clean and dry may be sufficient for them to heal.

CHAPTER FIFTEEN

Sexually Transmitted Skin Conditions

Since many of the S.T.D.s are acquired through skin contact, it's not surprising that these infections tend to affect the skin itself; or, the skin *plus* certain internal genital organs.

In enumerating those skin infections that are commonly linked to sexual contacts, the first and most serious would be syphilis. Gonorrhea can also be numbered among the S.T.D.s that can produce skin lesions; and, of course, herpes—both types—affects the skin. Then there are the venereal warts, which are very common and unsightly.

Pubic lice and scabies are also sometimes exchanged for the joys of sex. In other countries, principally those with low hygienic standards, chancroid, which resembles the chancre of syphilis, is a common skin disorder.

Syphilis & Gonorrhea Can Leave Their Mark

Syphilis was described and discussed in detail in Chapter 8. I will merely review, at this point, some facts on what this classic venereal disease does to the skin.

The earliest lesion is often on the skin. In contrast to herpes, which has a short incubation period—it ranges from a few days to two weeks—the chancre of syphilis takes its times and usually appears after some four to six weeks, although the range is wider than that. The chancre can appear in *less* than four weeks; or it can take as long as *ten* weeks to show up. As I have said, the sore isn't sore—it doesn't hurt. There may be one single lesion or possibly two; rarely are there more than that. The size varies greatly but in most cases it's a little smaller than a dime, and that includes the reddened area surrounding it. Most of the skin problems with syphilis occur in the secondary stage when all sorts of rashes can appear, all over the body. (Again, this is described in Chapter 8.)

Gonorrhea, too, can leave its mark. While skin problems arising from this disease are not frequently seen, they do occur. The eruptions look like little pus pimples, not very different from those seen in acne, which most often appear on the face. However, gonorrhea eruptions are usually in places on the body that acne bypasses: around the genital area, on the hands, or near the anus, although they are not limited to these areas. If they're in the early stages, lab tests can usually separate gonococcal from other lesions; and if they *are* gonococcal, they will usually respond well and quickly to antibiotic treatment.

Venereal Warts

There are a variety of names for venereal warts: genital warts, moist warts, and condyloma (acuminata). Their appearance is somewhat different from warts on the fingers inasmuch as they are usually softer, pink or reddish, and are often moist. Their location can be anywhere in the genital area but they are also common in the anal region among homosexual men. They may appear either singly, in a group of two or three, or in a cluster of so many that they will produce a cauliflower appearance. They tend to grow more rapidly in women, particularly in the presence of a discharge, or during pregnancies.

Syphilis is also capable of producing something that looks like a wart, but in *that* disease the "warts" are much broader based and are usually accompanied by other symptoms of the disease.

Genital warts are caused by the human papilloma virus. If they are located on the cervix, they can produce lesions that look like carcinoma. A biopsy is needed to determine what they are. This virus is suspected of being one of many agents that can trigger cancer of the cervix.

Genital warts can be treated by the person affected but it's best for a physician to do the treating because the drug (podophyllum) has to be applied locally, and great care is necessary to prevent injury to the surrounding skin. It should not be used during pregnancies. Other treatment methods exist, and sometimes surgical excision becomes necessary. However, none of the treatments is entirely satisfactory for all cases.

Herpes

The second chapter of this book deals with various aspects of herpes and I don't want to repeat all that information here. (See pp. 23-35). No section dealing with skin conditions that are sexually transmitted can fail to make some mention of herpes. Suffice to say here that it has become the most common of all the skin conditions that are sexually transmitted; that it's the most persistent; that it afflicts millions of Americans; and that, except for its first appearance, it is not generally confused with any of the other skin eruptions. Unlike other skin diseases, it tends to recur in the same spot, over and over again.

Pubic Lice

Strangely, the head louse and the crab louse each seeks its own turf: the former shuns the hair around the pubic area and the latter avoids the head. They are two different animals.

The crab louse is usually transmitted sexually, although there are many exceptions. This is one of the few sexually transmitted diseases that you *can* get from infested bedding, borrowed swim trunks, and—theoretically, at least—even from toilets, although I find this to be an unlikely source. I do, however, see many cases of crab lice on travelers returning from North Africa, Pakistan, Haiti, and other areas where hotel bedding may be infested.

Despite the fact that the crab lice are large and usually make their presence known in great numbers, it's not easy to see them with the naked eye. Their color is grayish. One way to get them for examination purposes is to press some scotch tape against the itchy pubic area; they will adhere to the tape. The eggs attach themselves to the hair, close to the skin. Upon examination of someone experiencing a bout of pubic lice, the scratchmarks made by the host bearer are more evident than the lice themselves, and these scratches often become infected.

A cure for pubic lice can readily be achieved by using one of several commercially available products, such as *Rid* or *Kwell*. Kwell requires a prescription, Rid does not. Directions must be strictly adhered to in order to avoid overtreatment, which usually occurs because the itch outlives the lice.

Scabies: A Mite That Causes A Mighty Itch

Although scabies occurs everywhere in the world, it's more common among the unwashed. In the late seventies, we experienced an epidemic of scabies that, for unknown reasons, subsided after several years. At present, it's rare in the U.S.

Scabies is caused by a little mite, a relative of the tick. Strictly speaking, it's not in the category of sexually transmitted diseases, but since it's often transmitted during the close contact of cohabitation, it seems appropriate to include it in this chapter.

The mite is too tiny to be seen with the naked eye, but it can be seen with a magnifying glass. Even then, it is more likely that one will see only the ducts through which the mite burrows.

The itch experienced with scabies not only interferes with sleep, but the irritation can become almost unbearable—much worse than the discomfort caused by crab lice. There are some effective drugs available for its treatment but, again, it's advisable to follow directions strictly and not to overtreat. Sufferers often do overtreat because the itch outlasts the infestation. The most effective preparations require a prescription because their excessive use must be avoided.

Chancroid—A Caution For The World Traveler

Chancroid is rarely acquired in the United States or Canada, but it is common in other countries. The disease produces ulcers in the genital region, resembling the chancre of syphilis. But chancroid is painful, and the base of the ulcer is softer than the syphilitic chancre. Like herpes and unlike syphilis, the incubation time for this disease, which is caused by a bacillus (Haemophylus ducreyi), is short—between four and six days.

Chancroid is sometimes mistaken for a severe case of herpes, particularly if the blister breaks and the infection produces a painful and confluent ulcer. Unlike the herpes lesion, which heals itself in a week or so, the chancroid progresses unless it's treated vigorously.

When someone is infected with chancroid, the lymph nodes in the groin are likely to become large and painful, more so than in a severe case of herpes. Effective treatment is available, but medical care is needed for proper diagnosis, selection of the right drug, and persistence in carrying out the treatment.

In this and other chapters I've described some of the sores and ulcers that make their appearance on the skin in the genital area. In my clinical experience, I have found that over a third of all genital ulcers seen nowadays are due to herpes. Five to ten percent are caused by syphilis. Some fifteen percent of the patients who have skin eruptions in the genital area are suffering from fungal infections. Chancroid is rare; so are granuloma inguinale and an ulcerated "molluscum contagiosum," an infection common among children.

The rest of what we see clinically represents widely scattered skin ailments ranging from psoriasis to non-specific infections, which means that it is unclear whether the bacteria found in an ulcer really caused it, or whether the bacteria are there because the ulcer provided them with a good breeding ground.

A scratch can often develop into a sore. Minor wounds from human bites can also lead to infection, and such wounds do not usually heal easily.

AIDS may first manifest itself with purplish skin lesions peculiar to this infection. More on this in Chapter 18.

CHAPTER SIXTEEN

Contraception and S.T.D.s

With growing knowledge about contraception and wider availability of various contraceptive devices, a greater range of women today are prepared for premarital and extramarital sex. But while the pill, the I.U.D., and other contraceptive methods temporarily lessened inhibitions, along with fear of pregnancy, they have done nothing to prevent the spread of S.T.D.s.

Before the newer contraceptive methods were developed, the two principal devices used to prevent pregnancy were the diaphragm and the condom, and it was the condom that did an excellent job of preventing the transmission of the venereal diseases. The condom, however, lost popularity alongside the newer methods, and from the point of view of spreading S.T.D.s, that's too bad. Fortunately, it is now regaining its deserved place among contraceptive methods.

The Pill, The I.U.D., And S.T.D.s

While the pill, by itself, cannot lead to a sexually transmitted disease, there is some indication—unconfirmed by appropriate medical studies—that the use of the pill affects the mucous lining of the vagina and makes it a more favorable environment for certain micro-organisms, such as monilia.

The I.U.D. neither prevents nor encourages the acquisition of a sexually transmitted disease. By providing a ladder on which bacteria from the vagina can reach the upper genital tract, an I.U.D. can, on rare occasions, lead to infections of the womb and to P.I.D. Such infections, however, would not be S.T.D.s. Douching by a woman wearing an I.U.D., if done at all, should be done gently and with minimal water pressure.

The Condom And S.T.D.s

Condoms are simple to use, inexpensive, easily available, and comparatively effective in the prevention of S.T.D.s. They offer dual protection against diseases and pregnancy and, even though they are less popular than other forms of contraceptives, billions of them are sold annually in this country.

Condoms are ordinarily made of latex, although there is also one very expensive type made from the gut of lambs. These materials are thin, strong, and elastic. They come in a choice of transparent or opaque; colored or plain; with or without reservoirs at the end; and can be had dry or prelubricated with silicone or other water-soluble substances. They come rippled, strictured, or contoured in various shapes.

The origin of this penile sheath is attributed to a French military doctor, Colonel Condom, after whom it is named.

Often, the condom is called a "rubber" or a "prophylactic;" and sometimes it's referred to as a "sheath," "French letter," "protective," "skin," or "safe."

While condom failure can happen, such accidents, which are the result of rupture or tears in the latex, are rare. There are two techniques that can help prevent such tears: if the condom is plain-ended, it should be unrolled in such a manner as to leave a half inch of space at the tip to accommodate the sperm fluid; and, it should be lubricated. However, the lubrication should be with vaginal cream or jelly—not petroleum jelly or Vaseline® since they can adversely affect the latex.

Preventing S.T.D.s With Other Contraceptive Methods

There are contraceptive jellies on the market, available without prescription, that can be used with or without a diaphragm. Such preparations, as well as others formulated as foams, gels, or vaginal suppositories, offer moderate protection against gonorrhea but there are no studies proving their usefulness against other S.T.D.s. Even in the case of gonorrhea, they are unreliable when used for this purpose. Some of the popular foams, creams, and jellies are: Crescent Cream or Jelly (Milex), Emko Foam, and Koromex Foam, Cream, or Jelly.

CHAPTER SEVENTEEN

S.T.D.s in the Gay Community

An estimated 3 to 5 percent of the men in this country are exclusively homosexual. Another 10 percent are bi-sexual, with their homosexual activities ranging from rare to occasional. Many more have isolated homosexual experiences but remain heterosexual throughout their lives.

It is important for clinicians to know a patient's sexual habits because the prevalence and types of infections we would expect and look for in gay men could be different from those usually found in heterosexuals. The most common of these infections are listed below.

There has been far less medical study and experience with lesbians than with gay males; so, obviously, we know much less about the former group than the latter. However, we do know that lesbians, as a group, have the lowest rate of S.T.D.s while gay men have, by far, the highest. This is attributed to the fact that gay males, although they frequently have long-lasting relationships, have, in the past, generally shown greater promiscuity than other population segments. This is neither a criticism nor a morality judgment—it's just a fact that is reaffirmed by the many thousands of gay men who visit our public health clinics. Any such fact is a group statistic and should not be applied to an individual. As with all group statistics, there are always many individual exceptions. In recent years, however, we have seen major changes taking place in the lifestyles of many gay men.

Types And Frequency Of S.T.D.s Found In Gay Males

The most common S.T.D.s generally found in all groups are also prevalent in homosexuals. But some diseases ordinarily found in the intestinal tract, where they have been acquired through food, can be transmitted sexually by gay men when they have anal intercourse.

In descending order of the incidence with which they occur, the most common infections among gay males are gonorrhea, non-specific urethritis, chlamydia, herpes, infections with pubic lice (pediculosis), venereal warts, syphilis, scabies, and hepatitis B. (Most of these are discussed in detail in other parts of this book. The *Index* will help you find the pages on which there is specific reference to them.)

Among other organisms that gay men can sexually transmit during anal intercourse we find amoeba and giardia. These are larger, one-celled organisms that we have found to be quite prevalent in recent years. Of course, it's also possible that we now test for the prevalence of organisms that we didn't formerly look for, and this could distort the apparent upward curve of frequency. We also see shigella and salmonella that

138

have been sexually transmitted during anal intercourse. These, too, are gastro-intestinal ailments that are ordinarily transmitted through food or by food handlers. Obviously, these bacteria are now finding new ports of entry into the body.

An Explanation For The High Incidence Of S.T.D.s Among Gays

No one can question the fact that a large number of sexual contacts increases the likelihood of picking up an S.T.D. This is true whether one is heterosexual or homosexual. However, gay males (and once again, let me say that I'm talking of group statistics and there are many individual exceptions) often report that they consummate sexual relations with people who are virtual strangers—often anonymous strangers. People met in gay bars, in gay baths, in public parks, and sometimes even in public restrooms, may become sex partners. These are usually fleeting relationships between people who have never met before and will never meet again after the isolated encounter. It's obvious that a man, under such circumstances, has no way of knowing what his momentary sex partner has brought to the mating, other than a mutual interest in the brief activity.

Many gay men visiting our clinics say quite honestly that they can't get in touch with their sexual contacts in order to urge them to get treatment, because they simply don't know the whereabouts, or sometimes even the names of people with whom they've had sexual relations. This factor has public health consequences inasmuch as it becomes impossible to trace back the chain of a communicable disease to its source. Efforts to stem the spread of an S.T.D. can be hampered by such anonymity. It has been estimated that the likelihood of exposure to an S.T.D. in the course of one night's visit to a gay bathhouse is one in three. For this reason, bathhouses have been closed in some communities.

Signs Of Rectal Gonorrhea

The information about gonorrhea in Chapter 7 applies, of course, to everyone, whatever his or her sexual proclivity. But special concern is directed to rectal gonorrhea in this chapter.

An infection in this organ of the body could show no signs at all; or there could be signs which could also be symptomatic of some ailments entirely unrelated to a venereal disease. This book is not meant to be a medical encyclopedia—and since I would not recommend that a man try to diagnose his own rectal ailment, there's not much point in listing all the possibilities. However, to give you some idea of why medical expertise should be sought for a proper diagnosis, let me say that the symptoms could be indicative of everything from internal or external hemorrhoids or an anal fissure to squamous cell carcinoma or anal cryptitis.

The uncharacteristic symptoms that might or might not be caused by the gonococcus could be any of these: a feeling of moistness, pain in conjunction with constipation or diarrhea, urgency to have a bowel movement, burning, or a discharge of blood or pus. All of these could be unrelated to an S.T.D., but someone with such symptoms should get a diagnosis through a physical examination that includes pertinent lab tests.

The examining physician has to use his or her judgment in deciding which tests are indicated. He or she may wish to have a culture done for gonorrhea, smears for amoebae, possibly a culture for chlamydia. If the doctor has reason to suspect the possibility of giardia, he or she might want to examine stool samples. If hepatitis is considered a possibility, blood serum tests would be performed. All of these tests require a wait of several days before the lab results are in. None of the tests is painful. They range in price from ten to fifty dollars, sometimes more, depending upon what test it is and what part of the country you live in. As with everything else, medical costs escalate in those parts of the country where the cost of living is higher.

Hepatitis B In Gay Males

There are three types of viral hepatitis. They are called A, B, and non-A, non-B. The reason for this third, somewhat vague name is that, at present, it is possible, by testing, to identify Type A and Type B. The third type is known to be a form of hepatitis but its characteristics are not clearly defined and do not always present a picture of sufficient clarity for medicine to designate it as "Type C." We know merely that it is hepatitis; and that it is neither Type A nor B. The only thing these three illnesses have in common is their preference for liver cells as a nesting place. Aside from that, the viruses are unrelated.

Hepatitis B, which used to be called serum hepatitis, is the type we're talking about in this chapter because we see much of it in the gay, male population. (The other types are covered in greater detail on pp. 101-103.) In the past, it was believed that this infection was transmitted principally through blood and infected needles used by drug addicts. While such needles do, indeed, serve as transmitters, it has also been found that this virus is present in both saliva and semen, and that it is commonly transmitted through these media.

Any sexual activity that would put you in contact with the saliva or semen of someone suffering from hepatitis B would open the door to such an infection. However, there are other ways of passing it along.

Hepatitis B is also transmitted through the blood. This can occur with transfusions; when health professionals or others accidentally prick themselves with a needle that is contaminated with the virus; or by injecting drugs into the blood stream with an unclean needle.

Hepatitis A is most commonly transmitted through the stools. Food handlers who have this disease and do not follow good hygiene practices (including washing their hands thoroughly with soap and water after going to the bathroom) can pass along hepatitis A. What puts this disease into a book on the S.T.D.s is the fact that a man engaging in anal intercourse with someone whose stools carry the virus is also likely to pick up the infection.

When symptoms develop—and they don't always—they are usually a combination of fatigue and lassitude. In a mere ten percent of all cases, jaundice occurs—a yellow discoloration of the whites of the eyes, the skin, and the fingernails. Most cases are mild and only one percent require hospitalization. Some are followed by chronic liver disorders. A few may progress rapidly and prove deadly.

Once someone has experienced this disease, there is immunity for life against new infections with the *same* hepatitis virus. Unfortunately, this immunity does not extend to *other* types of hepatitis. There is a blood test that can tell if one has hepatitis B—or has had it. Since most people don't know if or when they have it, the results of such a test sometimes come as a surprise. Those who are infected and aren't aware of it can transmit the infection for long periods of time, sometimes for years, through their saliva, blood, or sperm.

One protection against hepatitis B is the condom. There is also an effective vaccine available but it is, so far, rather expensive. Anybody who is gay, sexually active, and able to afford this vaccine might want to discuss this with his treating physician.

More details on hepatitis are to be found in Chapter 10, on pages 97-103.

Salmonella, Shigella, Giardia, And Amoebic Infections

These infections usually cause gastro-intestinal symptoms, often diarrhea. They can also produce fever and general malaise. Giardia infections tend to be prolonged. Intermittent bellyaches or vague discomfort in the abdominal region are common symptoms, as are tiredness, weight loss, and a tendency to anemia. Once the cause of these symptoms is determined, however, treatment with a drug called Metronidazole is relatively simple and quite effective.

Salmonella and shigella infections are usually short-lived, with acute intestinal symptoms (diarrhea, nausea, cramps, and fever) that may last a few days, often clearing up without medication. There are literally hundreds of foods that can become infected with salmonella and shigella bacteria, including two that aren't usually thought of by laypersons when they try to determine "what they ate" that might have caused the problem. These two are fowl and fish—either of which, if insufficiently cooked, can implant such an infection. But, as I said, there are hundreds of foods, perhaps thousands, that could be the culprits. Ordinarily, these would be considered G-I infections, but since they are in the intestinal tract, they can lodge in the stools and the rectum—which puts them into the category of diseases that can be sexually transmitted.

The amoeba is a different kettle of bug. Some low-grade infections of amoeba can go unnoticed for long periods of time. Sooner or later, however, the person with amebiasis may experience recurrent bouts of diarrhea and stomach cramps, sometimes alternating with constipation. The stools would tend to be soft and could contain flecks of blood-stained mucous. In rare, severe cases, there could be blood in the stools accompanied by fatigue to the point of exhaustion.

If the liver is involved, and it can be, then the right, upper side of the abdomen may be painful and very tender to the touch. The liver can be affected by amebiasis without any signs of diarrhea or other intestinal disturbances. One of the ways a physician can confirm a suspicion of liver involvement is to take a blood sample and have serological tests for amebiasis performed.

For all of the infections discussed in this section, lab tests are available to determine which type of invader has made its entry into the body. Once the type of organism has been identified, the appropriate course of treatment can be recommended. Sometimes, no treatment at all is indicated.

Importance Of Medical Checkups For The Gay Male

The probability of acquiring an S.T.D. is proportional to the number of exposures and to the amount of risk-taking with unknown partners. While a monogamous gay man need not exercise any more precautions than his heterosexual counterpart who is also monogamous, a man with many sexual contacts—whatever his proclivity—should seek medical diagnosis if he shows any suggestive symptoms. Once again, I would emphasize that a gay male serves his own best interests when he tells his physician or clinician that he is a practicing homosexual. This information enables the doctor to use the appropriate tests from the appropriate locations in the body.

Among the various tests that might be performed, the most important are the blood tests for AIDS and syphilis (see Chapter 8 on *Syphilis,* and Chapter 18 on *AIDS*), followed by tests for gonococci. These would be smear and bacteriological cultures from the penis, rectum, and throat.

Other tests are less useful as routine procedures but may be indicated just the same, depending on the symptoms. For example, an infection with gonococcal or non-gonococcal urethritis is self-evident—anyone suffering this illness would be likely to seek medical care. The same refers to pediculosis, scabies, and venereal warts. Herpes is also self-evident but since we have not yet come up with a satisfactory treatment for it, making a diagnosis is less critical than with gonorrhea or syphilis. On the other hand, a diagnosis of herpes eliminates the worry that a lesion could be due to syphilis. This could provide some measure of mental relief, if one can say that there is any "relief" attached to having herpes.

CHAPTER EIGHTEEN

AIDS

Acquired Immunodeficiency Syndrome

AIDS is a sexually transmissible infection caused by a virus. This infection may produce no symptoms at all for many years, perhaps never. On the other hand, after an incubation period that can range from months to years, the virus may cause a disease characterized by a loss of immunity against micro-organisms that pose little or no threat to people whose immune systems are intact. Consequently, the outward symptoms of AIDS are not those of the AIDS infection itself, but of other infections that are acquired because the body's natural resistance to them has been lost.

The AIDS Virus

The virus that causes AIDS is named HIV, *human immunodeficiency virus*. Several closely related types of HIV have been identified, but this fact is, at present, of more scientific than practical interest.

Another name for the same virus—an older name—is HTLV-III/LAV, which stands for *Human T-lymphotropic virus, type III/lymphadenopathy associated virus*. "T-lymphotropic" refers to the fact that it affects a certain part of the human lymphatic system. "Lymphadenopathy associated virus" is abbreviated to "LAV." For reasons of simplicity, the term HIV was recently adopted.

There is much controversy about the origin of this infection, which is new to mankind. One link, considered to be speculative at this time, is that the virus is closely related to one found in monkeys and perhaps other animal species, and that, somehow, it accidentally crossed over to humans, perhaps as the result of a person being bitten by an infected animal. Once it invaded humans, it underwent slight mutations and remains, like most viruses, subject to further changes.

Micro-organisms invading our bodies have their favorite target organs. The tuberculosis bacillus prefers the lungs, the hepatitis virus likes to nest in the liver, other viruses prefer the brain, causing encephalitis, and so on. The AIDS virus chooses the lymphatic system primarily, the system essential to maintaining our immune mechanism. This renders the affected person unprotected against organisms which the body ordinarily can fend off. The immunodeficiency caused by such a damaged lymphatic system can produce a wide variety of secondary illnesses.

Groups Infected by AIDS

Male homosexuals and bisexuals still account for the largest percentage of AIDS cases, close to 75 percent. While the overall number of AIDS cases continues to increase, the *percentage* of male homosexuals and bisexuals who are infected is decreasing.

In the U.S., there are still about twelve times as many males as females who are afflicted. In Africa, by contrast, the ratio is close to one to one. Intravenous drug abusers are the second largest group, particularly if their numbers include homosexual drug users.

One to two percent of AIDS occurs in each of these groups: persons with hemophilia, persons who had blood transfusions before tests for AIDS became available in March 1985, and infants born to infected mothers. Four percent of the cases have been attributed to viruses spread through heterosexual intercourse.

Some 5 percent of AIDS patients cannot be categorized, but it is believed that transmission occurred in one of the abovementioned ways.

The spread of this infection is gaining speed and, by now, AIDS is a global problem, with close to a hundred countries reporting cases. While the U.S. still reports the vast majority of cases, the reliability of reporting systems varies greatly from country to country. We do know that in some African regions, a larger percentage of the population is infected than in the U.S.

Full-blown cases of AIDS—those who are obviously sick—represent only a small part of the problem. It is estimated that one to two million people in the United States are already infected with the HIV virus, half of them heterosexuals. Based on our present, limited experience, we estimate that about a third of these people eventually will develop AIDS.

Pneumocystis Carinii And Kaposi's Sarcoma

In those infected persons in whom the disease progresses, one or both of two rare diseases appear: a kind of pneumonia caused by the pneumocystis carinii, a parasitic infection of the lungs; and a type of cancer known as Kaposi's Sarcoma. These two diseases are not found in all AIDS cases but do occur in more than 80 percent of them.

Kaposi's Sarcoma (KS) can occur anywhere on the surface of the skin or in the mouth. In early stages, it may look like a bruise or a blue-violet or brownish spot. The spot or spots persist and may grow larger. KS can also spread to internal organs.

Early Symptoms Of An AIDS Infection

Most individuals infected with the AIDS virus have no symptoms and feel well. Others, not long after the infection, develop a mild, flu-like illness of short duration. After varying periods of time, which could be months or years, some infected people develop symptoms that do not necessarily point to AIDS and could be ascribed to a number of causes. Such symptoms may include fatigue, slight fever, loss of appetite and weight, diarrhea, and night sweating.

The pneumocystis carinii pneumonia has symptoms similar to any other form of severe pneumonia—in particular, coughing, difficulty in breathing, and fever. The cough is rather dry with no phlegm accompanying it.

Because of the body's impaired immunity, other infectious organisms may take advantage of the lack of resistance. Such infections are called "opportunistic." It appears that microorganisms, with which a person with an intact immune system can usually cope, make the most of any opportunity where they can gain the upper hand. These infections include unusually severe yeast and other fungal infections, cytomegalovirus, the herpes virus, and parasites such as Toxoplasma or Cryptosporidia, as well as many others. Mild infections with these organisms do not suggest immune deficiency.

Diagnosing AIDS

The diagnosis of a fully developed case of AIDS poses no difficulty. In contrast to most other diseases, however, AIDS may have many different manifestations, depending on a variety of "opportunistic" infections. Conversely, it can have no symptoms or signs at all—or anything in between these two extremes.

The diagnosis of the actual disease AIDS is usually made on clinical grounds, meaning from the combination of (a) a patient's history, (b) the symptoms, and (c) certain blood tests which can demonstrate damage to some types of white blood cells. A positive blood test showing the presence of the HIV virus in the body also helps in the diagnosis.

The most certain test for a definite diagnosis would be to grow and identify the virus by culture method. But this approach is difficult, time consuming, expensive, and very few places are equipped to grow the virus. Aside from such culturing, there is no single, definitive blood test for AIDS. Any test that looks for the presence of antibodies to the HIV virus in the blood has to be confirmed by other tests before being accepted as diagnostically correct. (Antibodies are substances produced by the body in an attempt to fight off invading organisms. Various tests can reveal their presence in the blood serum, indicating that such an invasion has taken place.)

A positive blood test, confirmed by other tests, and combined with a patient history and physical examination, can usually resolve a questionable case.

For practical purposes, the presence of Kaposi's sarcoma and pneumocystis pneumonia—in the absence of any known cause of immune deficiency—means that the patient has AIDS.

AIDS cases are classified in four groups, according to the stage of the disease. Group I includes patients with vague and usually mild symptoms similar to a flu or mononucleosis—with such symptoms appearing shortly after the time of infection. Were a blood test to be taken at this point, it would not necessarily show a positive reaction.

Group II comprises those with no symptoms but with positive blood tests. This is, by far, the largest group. Millions fall into this segment of AIDS cases.

Group III is made up of those who have, in addition to positive blood tests, persistent, generalized swelling of their lymph nodes.

Group IV comprises those with the overt disease and showing any, or several of the symptoms described above.

More About Blood Tests For AIDS

The various antibody tests in the blood are used not only to diagnose, but to screen and to test donated blood and plasma in order to help prevent transmission of AIDS from blood transfusions or the use of blood products. Patients with hemophilia depend on such blood products and were at particular risk before serological tests were developed that can screen out blood that tests positive for AIDS.

For anyone interested in having his or her blood examined, screening tests are available through private physicians and most state and many local health departments. If the doctor or health department contacted does not perform the test, they can usually refer one to an appropriate testing source—with the assurance of confidentiality.

You may want to know what "testing" involves. In brief, it first involves the use of a procedure that employs enzymes to search for antibodies in the blood. Should this test prove negative, nothing further is done unless there is strong suspicion of an infection. On the other hand, if the results are positive, the enzyme test has to be corroborated before it is accepted. At least one confirmatory test is then performed, usually one called the Western Blot Assay Test. Only if both tests are positive does one assume the presence of an AIDS infection.

On Being A Carrier

There is a vast difference between having a confirmed, positive blood test for the HIV virus and having the disease AIDS.

Though most people who test positive are asymptomatic, feeling well and normal, they are carriers of the AIDS virus. In some cases, the infection does progress, but it's difficult to state how many carriers will actually develop AIDS because the percentage varies from group to group. However, our statistics at this time indicate that, within five years, about 5 to 10 percent of those who test positive will develop the disease

AIDS. In another 25 percent, the infection may manifest itself in the form of an "AIDS related complex" (ARC), which consists mostly of persistent, multiple swelling of lymph nodes. The other two-thirds will be well after five years.

We don't know why some people develop the disease AIDS early on, while other positive carriers remain in apparent good health. Much hope is pinned on finding the factor or factors that help determine this. Some believe that stress, drug abuse, and other infections—particularly sexually transmitted diseases—weaken the immune system and facilitate the progression from a latent to an active state. Because the asymptomatic period can last so long, there is always hope that a drug will be developed in time to avert progression from the carrier stage to the symptomatic phase.

There are some practical difficulties for the perfectly well person who reacts positively to the HIV virus. Though not suffering from the disease AIDS, he or she, as a carrier of the virus, can transmit it to others through sexual contact. Some states are considering the possibility of requiring a blood test for AIDS for people applying for a marriage license. Some businesses, government agencies, and insurance companies have been trying to erect barriers discriminating against those who are well, but infected—although many state legislatures are trying to protect this huge population segment against such mandated tests.

One important question for those who may have been exposed to the AIDS virus sexually or through I.V. drug abuse is how long it takes for the blood serum to show the presence of antibodies—that is, to test positively if infection has taken place. This period has not been determined precisely; it, too, seems to vary greatly. We know that it can be only a few weeks after infection or as long as six months later. But after a year, almost anyone who has been infected will develop antibodies, which will show up in a serology test.

The Treatment Of AIDS

Until 1986, no treatment was available that could affect the AIDS virus or reverse the damage it causes to the immune system. Standard therapy has been—and still is—to treat aggressively any acquired infections as they occur.

The search for anti-viral drugs is being pressed vigorously, and a number of them are under study. Some drugs have been found to inhibit the AIDS virus. One in particular, *Retrovir,* has already been approved by the Food and Drug Administration (FDA) for use by prescription.

Retrovir (the generic name is *Zidovudine*—formerly called AZT, which stands for azidothymidine) interferes with the reproduction of the HIV virus and has been shown to prolong the lives of some AIDS and ARC (AIDS related complex) sufferers. The supply of the drug is still limited but this shortage should be alleviated soon. For cases deemed suitable for treatment with Retrovir, the drug has to be obtained through a pharmacy and requires a physician's prescription. So far, Retrovir has not been approved for *all* manifestations of AIDS. Despite its speedy approval by the FDA, this drug has been associated with occasional, serious side effects. Among these are a suppression of the bone marrow, leading to anemia or a very low white blood cell count. Retrovir shares this adverse reaction with many other powerful drugs in common use for other illnesses. When such side effects occur, they usually necessitate blood transfusions, a reduction of the dose used, or interruption of the treatment. Long-term effects of the drug are not known as yet, nor do we have much experience concerning Retrovir's interaction with other drugs commonly used to treat opportunistic infections.

Other side effects, usually tolerable, include nausea and headaches, which are experienced by approximately half the treated patients, and such other minor problems as muscle pain.

Retrovir is not considered a cure for AIDS; but, so far, it has demonstrated that it can improve the survival period for certain patients with pneumocystis pneumonia and ARC (AIDS related complex). For the time being, it is a front-line drug, providing a treatment for many unknown factors associated with an AIDS infection. Thus, it is a significant milestone in our search for a treatment or cure for this disease. By no means is it a final milestone in the ongoing search for a breakthrough drug that will help control AIDS.

A major drawback is the high cost of Retrovir. Its manufacturer, Burroughs Wellcome, responds to comments about its high cost by pointing out that two-thirds of the patients treated with it are able to continue or resume productive lives and that the cost is substantially lower than the cost of treating AIDS patients who are *not* on this drug. In addition, the company justifies its price by quoting the high cost of production and the fact that it has already borne enormous up-front development costs of more than $80 million, without any assurance that the drug would ever reach the market. Still, the cost—about $10,000 a year per patient—is a major worry for patients and for hospitals, insurance companies, and other agencies involved in the care of AIDS patients.

Another drawback of the drug—certainly minor when compared to the disease itself—is that it must be taken on an empty stomach every four hours. Patients must set an alarm clock so that they will not forget to take the drug in the middle of the night, and they must schedule their food intake around the drug. Even when feeling quite well, they cannot enjoy the luxury of an occasional period when their sickness is not uppermost in their mind. While on Retrovir, they receive a sharp reminder of it six times a day. However, while the search for a better drug continues, patients are more than willing to undergo these hardships in exchange for the benefits Retrovir can deliver to some of them.

In addition to Retrovir, which was approved by the FDA in record time, there are at least eight other drugs in the trial stage that show some promise. One drug, DDC, under investigation at the Stanford University Medical Center, may have fewer side effects than Retrovir. Other drugs include Interferon alpha, Ribavirin, Interleukin-2, and Foscarnet.

Researchers are optimistic that it may become possible soon to arrest an early viral infection and hold it at bay. This would be particularly beneficial to the many people who are carriers but have not yet developed any symptoms.

A Vaccine For AIDS

An AIDS vaccine is not around the corner. Many approaches are under trial but researchers are confronted by huge problems. First, who wants to be a subject in a research project when any negative effect the injection of an experimental vaccine might have is unknown? Also, it is difficult to prove the effectiveness of a vaccine if it takes as long as five years, sometimes longer, from the time of exposure to develop the disease.

The difficulty of developing a vaccine is increased by the fact that, at this time, we don't even know how many different strains of the virus exist. The AIDS virus tends to mutate, so even after a vaccine is developed, we will need to continue to monitor its effectiveness. Despite all the obstacles, the need for a vaccine is so pressing that research, in this country and abroad, continues to have the highest of priorities.

One encouraging aspect of the search for a vaccine lies in the very fact that the virus does mutate. This raises a hope that sometime in the future, a less- or non-virulent strain might be found that could be used for immunizations, such as cowpox served to immunize against the virulent human smallpox.

Most vaccines are tried out first on animals, with the exception of those diseases like whooping cough and meningococcal meningitis, which do not affect animals. Only the chimpanzee has shown a reaction to the AIDS virus and chimps are an endangered species, as well as being very expensive to obtain. There are a small number of them here in the U.S. available for medical research but not enough for any valid conclusions to be drawn from vaccine studies in which the chimps are subjects. It appears likely that experiments will have to be carried out on human volunteers.

One such experiment is underway in Zaire, where the disease is much more prevalent than in the United States. This trial is being carried out by a French team. In the U.S., work is in progress at George Washington University and is also being done by some companies, including Bristol-Myers.

Jonas Salk, who produced the first polio vaccine, favors a "killed" vaccine rather than one that uses a live but much-weakened ("attenuated") virus. He feels that the former will be quicker to produce and safer to use. But any vaccine will face the difficult problems of finding volunteers, determining what type of volunteer to accept, and the ultimate decision on whether the vaccine is useful.

Even if and when researchers should have a vaccine available, they would need to decide which group in their study should get it and which group should act as a "control" group, receiving a placebo instead of the vaccine. From an ethical point of view, both groups would have to be indoctrinated in the dos and don'ts of AIDS prevention.

Although researchers may begin testing AIDS vaccines soon, a useful vaccine is unlikely to be available until the 1990s.

Blood Transfusions And The AIDS Virus

Hundreds of thousands of people who received blood transfusions between 1978 and 1985 may want to have their blood tested for the AIDS virus. Generally speaking, the risk for these persons is very low. However, it is higher for anyone who received a large number of transfusions, especially in areas of the U.S. where a high number of AIDS cases appeared prior to those transfusions. Such areas of greater early incidence include New York, San Francisco, Los Angeles, Houston, Miami, Washington, D.C., and Newark.

March 1985 marked the beginning of AIDS testing of donated blood. In the case of people who received transfusions before that date, their risk decreases as time goes on since the virus was not at all widespread before then. The risk of having received a transfusion with infected blood varies greatly and many people are sufficiently anxious about their own situation to want the reassurance they would get from a negative test. Within this group of people who had transfusions between 1978 and March 1985, the decision on whether to have a blood test is up to the individual. The major advantage of having such a test is that it offers peace of mind to those who test negative—and that would include the great majority of these people. Those whose blood proves positive would benefit from special AIDS counseling, usually available through state or local health departments. There are also some blood banks that can refer people to AIDS counselors.

Of course, as pointed out before, a positive blood test does not mean a diagnosis of AIDS. On the other hand, someone who tests positive, although never having experienced any symptoms of the disease, can still suffer tremendously from the emotional impact of this finding.

I also pointed out earlier in this chapter that one positive blood test is meaningless unless it is confirmed by a second, different type of test. Both must be positive before someone is considered infected. Even then a repeat of the tests may be indicated in some cases.

Of course, it is important for sexually active persons to know whether they are infected so that they are aware that they risk spreading the virus to their partners. It is also important for someone testing positive to inform his or her personal physician of this finding so that the right examinations can be performed should certain symptoms, such as coughing or diarrhea, develop. Knowing that a patient has tested positive for the AIDS virus would suggest to a physician the need to search for micro-organisms that would not be sought under ordinary circumstances.

In the U.S., the blood supply is strained by a declining number of donors and we can expect this supply to be taxed severely when the AIDS drug, Retrovir, is in wider use. Sooner or later, about a third of those receiving this drug require blood transfusions because, as mentioned earlier, one of its side effects is the development of anemia. Increased use of the drug will lead to heavy demands on the blood supply.

Because members of the gay community are at highest risk for AIDS, their blood is now refused by blood banks. Some gay leaders have indicated that they may set up special donation centers where healthy people in this group, non-reactors or those with negative test results, may donate blood specifically earmarked for use by AIDS sufferers. Unlike the second highest risk group, the I.V. drug users, the gay community is rather well organized and, should its members initiate the setting up of such centers, they could make a substantial contribution to helping those in need of transfusions.

On the subject of blood transfusions, there are two points that should be emphasized here. First, no one gets AIDS from *giving* blood. There is absolutely no danger of contracting the infection as a result of being a donor. All equipment used in blood banks is disposable and sterile. Since the need for blood is so acute, the public is urged to contribute to the blood banks in their community.

The second point, which can't be emphasized often enough, is that those who are in high risk groups, particularly those who have had homosexual experiences, even years ago, or used I.V. drugs, should not offer their blood. It would not be accepted in any event.

Transmission Of The AIDS Virus

In practically all cases, transmission of the AIDS virus takes place in one of two ways: through sexual contact with an infected partner; or through infected blood, which includes exposure of the fetus in the womb. Though theoretically possible, other methods of transmission play a negligible role.

This signifies that an AIDS epidemic is obviously different from influenza and the many upper respiratory epidemics, which are airborne; from intestinal infections, including hepatitis A, which are borne by food or water; or from infections transmitted by insects. Thus, AIDS *is* preventable, if certain specific, precautionary measures are taken.

Where transmission through blood is concerned, the widespread practice among drug users of sharing needles and syringes is the greatest contributing factor. Shared injection paraphernalia (dirty "works") provide the ideal means for the virus to be handed over from a carrier to one who is uninfected. A single incident is sufficient to achieve such a transfer.

Altering this custom of "sharing" could be a major factor in derailing the epidemic. Unfortunately, drug addicts as a group are difficult to reach and to reeducate. The majority of addicts have other things on their mind, such as getting their next fix, or raising the money for it. Although educational efforts are being directed at this population segment, drug users, in contrast to homosexuals, are suspicious of advice. Given a life replete with risks, the threat of AIDS seems remote to many drug users.

There is much discussion on the subject of introducing an exchange program for addicts—providing them with clean syringes and needles for the purpose of curbing the spread of AIDS. The effects of such a program are debatable; there are potential benefits and potential hazards in such an undertaking.

Supplying the "works" has been found in other countries to increase, rather than lessen the use of drugs. Those who use drugs occasionally, or who use them without injection, could escalate to injection, and to more frequent use, should the paraphernalia become easily available. But above and beyond this possibility is the fact that supplying needles and syringes appears to condone the injection of drugs, thus hindering the efforts of many groups to discourage this practice. There is also the fact that clean needles would have to be available at the crucial moment—immediately after the drug has been obtained. If not, any available needle, clean or dirty, will be used. Intravenous drug users are not known for their advance planning.

Apart from drug users, transfusions of whole blood or its components have been responsible in the past for passing along the AIDS virus. Much has been learned on this subject since the outbreak of AIDS, and two factors now guard against transfused blood becoming the means of transmission for the virus. First, donated blood is now tested for AIDS before it's used. Second, blood donations are not accepted from people in high risk groups. There was never any danger of getting AIDS because you donated blood. Donors have never been at risk.

Avoiding the sexual transfer of the AIDS virus requires a modification of behavior that sharply conflicts with the sexual freedom of the '60s and '70s, the height of the sexual revolution. Many groups, including bachelors and unmarried women, divorcees, and members of the gay community have, indeed, changed their lifestyles and become much more cautious about engaging in casual sexual relationships. However, as stated previously, most cases of sexually transmitted AIDS have occurred in the gay community. About 4 to 6 percent of all cases can be attributed to heterosexual intercourse, and this figure is on the rise.

Statistics from San Francisco and New York City comparing current sexual behavior in the gay community with the pre-AIDS era show that knowledge and fear of infection have brought about major changes in gay lifestyles.

There has been a 75 percent decrease in the number of "extra-domestic" sex partners—that is, new and sometimes casual relationships established through chance contacts. There has been a large decline in gay men's use of public bathhouses, which are being closed up in some communities. The use of condoms has increased from less than 2 percent to more than 20 percent. However, the incidence of sexual abstinence has not risen, except for individuals experiencing phases of acute illness.

Women And AIDS

The number of women who have AIDS is much smaller than the number of men. In terms of percentages, the sources of their infections differ from the male population. Approximately one-half of women with AIDS acquired it through drug abuse; the other half from male sex partners. The number of people in the latter group is rising faster than in any other group.

This rise in AIDS cases among women is a matter of major concern for two reason: first, women are at greater risk of acquiring AIDS through intercourse with an infected male than men are from women. The second concern is the rising incidence of AIDS in children, transmitted from their mothers, who may not show any outward sign of the disease.

The men who transmit AIDS to women are primarily I.V. drug users; secondarily, bisexuals; and, to a lesser extent, men who have been infected by other women.

Heterosexual contact is the only category of transmission in which women with AIDS outnumber men with AIDS. From a public health viewpoint, as well as that of the individuals involved, women should be aware of the risk of acquiring the infection through sexual intercourse and should adopt a risk-reducing lifestyle. Contraceptives brought about the sexual revolution; AIDS is responsible for the burgeoning counter-revolution where sex is concerned.

The fact is that the AIDS virus is not partial to homosexuals and I.V. drug users; it is a non-discriminating infector, willing to seize an opportunity when it presents itself. In a heterosexual relationship where the partners know little of each other's past sexual history, both people should be aware that the possibility of infection exists. It has been said, appropriately, that when you go to bed with someone you hardly know, you're going to bed with his (or her) whole sexual history.

Statistics show that the rate of infection among black and Hispanic women is comparatively high because their sex partners more frequently have a history of drug abuse.

Although she may not develop the disease itself, a woman whose blood serum shows that she is infected with the AIDS virus has to face major difficulties in her life. Nearly all such women are of child-bearing age and run the risk of infecting their fetus during pregnancy. A less justified fear is that they might infect their families. And, if single, they face the horrendous task of telling a new sex partner of their infection.

Now that the AIDS virus has been isolated, we know that it can be transmitted not only through blood and semen, but also through secretions from the cervix and vagina, as well as through menstrual blood. Thus heterosexual, vaginal sex is an obvious channel of transmission, both from men to women and from women to men.

Celibacy certainly prevents infection. Since this is an unrealistic expectation for people in their sexually active years, the best alternative is to use condoms during intercourse because they do block the passage of the virus. If condoms are used, their efficacy is increased when used in conjunction with spermicidal vaginal inserts that kill viruses. Nonoxynol

(Semicid) is one such spermicidal. Another suggestion for people concerned about AIDS is to engage in monogamous relationships, changing partners as infrequently as possible. Neither of these alternatives to celibacy is absolutely reliable in preventing the transmission of an AIDS infection—they are merely the best we have at the moment.

Increasingly, condom sales are being made to women; they are being targeted by condom manufacturers with ads in many of the women's magazines and through new packaging that no longer tries to convey a macho image to the buyer. In many drugstores, condoms are displayed next to feminine hygiene products. However, it is more often the man who has an aversion to condoms than the woman. Not only do many men dislike using them, but they become distrustful of a woman who suggests their use, suspecting that she might possibly be infected. This puts the woman in a double bind: at risk of infection if no condom is used and at risk of destroying a relationship if her suggestion that a condom be used is misinterpreted.

The subject of condoms has become a common topic of conversation among women, many of whom now feel that the use of these devices has shifted from contraception to AIDS prevention. In some circles, the concern among women has reached near-panic proportions, much more than during the herpes fright in the '70s. Evidence points to the fact that single women, while not turning to celibacy, have become more sexually selective.

Special difficulties are experienced by married women who learn that their husbands are, or were, bisexual or gay. It is estimated that approximately 25 percent of all homosexual men marry, at least for a short period of time—some to have children, many to gain societal approval.

For a woman, finding out that her husband is gay can be a tremendous shock, heightened immeasurably by the threat of AIDS. Many such marriages, by means of mutual accommodations, have survived in the past, particularly if children are involved. The AIDS threat makes this more difficult a situation to resolve, since by the time the wife learns her husband is gay or bisexual, marital sex has usually ceased. The likelihood of the wife's having been infected with AIDS depends on her husband's earlier lifestyle. Whether to have a serological test is a difficult personal decision that each woman has to make for herself.

Unless a woman comes to her physician with a story about her husband's gay or bisexual life, or the doctor knows a woman patient to be a drug user or prostitute, he will not ordinarily test for AIDS. Thus, the diagnosis of AIDS in women is usually delayed because there has been no reason to suspect that it might exist.

AIDS In Children

The number of children infected with the AIDS virus is growing ominously. It is estimated that they are being born at the rate of three thousand a year, many of them with no early signs of the disease. Their number is expected to continue to increase dramatically.

Women who know that they are carrying the virus, even though they have no symptoms and are apparently healthy, should defer pregnancy. If they do become pregnant, an abortion should be seriously considered. This viewpoint is shared even by some spokespersons who represent groups generally opposed to abortion.

If there is even the remotest possibility of exposure to the HIV virus, a pregnant woman would be well advised to have a test for infection early in her pregnancy, although she should not be required by law to do so. Such testing is done uniformly with assurance of confidentiality.

Children usually contract the infection from their mother before or during delivery. In the majority of cases, the mother was infected by a drug user or bisexual male partner, or is an I.V. drug user herself.

Infants can also acquire the AIDS infection through breast milk. If a substitute donor for breast milk is used, it is a good idea to screen her blood for HIV.

Among the many problems that arise in the care of HIV positive children is the dilemma concerning their attendance at day care centers, kindergartens and schools. The generally accepted view is that they should attend if they are asymptomatic. However, the situation is different if they are symptomatic, so the decision has to be made on a case-by-case basis.

There is also the question of whether a child's infection should be kept confidential. It is helpful for the teacher to be made aware of it; however, this should be done only with the full consent of the parent or guardian.

Screening of healthy children for HIV infections before admitting them to day care centers or schools should not be done. If an otherwise healthy child is known to be a positive reactor, others should not be informed of this fact unless the child's parent or guardian wants the information to become public and consents to its dissemination.

Because the households of drug addicts are not the choice environment in which children should be brought up, foster homes are often sought for HIV positive children if either parent has a drug problem. However, finding a foster home for such a child is extremely difficult. Whenever possible, an HIV infected child should remain, if not with its own parents, then with grandparents or other branches of the extended family.

Treating children, particularly small children and infants who have AIDS, is very difficult since their response to presently available drugs is less likely to delay the progress of the disease than would be the case in an adult. Often, the available drugs fail when used on children. Once it becomes symptomatic, the course of the AIDS infection in a child tends to be more rapid.

Among all these bleak and perplexing factors there is one that holds forth more promise: a positive blood test for AIDS in a newborn or in a child less than fifteen months old may merely be due to the transmission of maternal antibodies (substances in the blood that attempt to fight the AIDS virus) without infection with the virus itself. In such cases, the positive blood test will gradually fade and become negative after the age of fifteen months.

For this reason, it is essential to repeat serological tests in small children, unless they develop AIDS-related symptoms. After this fifteen-month period, a positive test in a child means that it has been exposed to the virus and infected, usually by the mother.

Often, both parents of a child with an HIV infection are seemingly perfectly healthy, and the child may be the first person in the family to develop symptoms of AIDS. In such cases, all possible risk factors in both parents have to be explored. To prevent such cases, there should be an expansion of HIV antibody testing for pregnant women, always with voluntary consent and with assurance of confidentiality.

At present, no one is proposing mandatory testing of pregnant women. If done, the testing should be performed as early as possible in the pregnancy and—depending on circumstances and the environment—repeated several months after the first test.

Mandatory premarital testing is considered ineffective in reducing HIV infections. However, sperm donors for artificial insemination should be tested both initially and repeatedly.

AIDS Children And Immunizations

The usual immunization of children against common childhood diseases presents a special problem for those infected with the AIDS virus. Generally speaking, it is all right for them to receive "inactivated" or "killed" vaccines, such as those against diphtheria, tetanus, whooping cough, and polio (the Salk vaccine). However, they should not be immunized with live vaccines that produce an attenuated or mild form of the disease. This latter group would include immunizations for measles, German measles, mumps, and polio (with the oral vaccine).

Educating Children About AIDS

No one really knows the answer to this question: At what age, and to what extent, should children be educated about AIDS? There are many opinions on this subject and common sense should prevail. It is doubtful that elementary school children would understand the dangers of contracting AIDS and ways to prevent it. After elementary school, the subject of sex education and, in particular, AIDS information, is still a delicate matter; many people believe that the responsibility lies with the parents. Unfortunately, most parents are so uninformed or misinformed about this disease that at home education is not practical. Informing children in school is also difficult as it requires knowledge, skill, tact, and sensitivity, and most teachers feel unqualified to handle the subject.

One school of thought favors an educational approach that recommends total sexual abstinence, with emphasis on the dangers of premarital sex. While this may be valid as an *option* for young people, it would need to be included along with *other* options in a broader approach to the whole subject of premarital sex, contraception, and prevention of disease. The controversy is reminiscent of the old maxim, "Be good; and if you can't be good, be careful."

I believe that high school students should learn about the common ways viral transmission occurs, as well as the preventive measures that are available.

How To Avoid Getting AIDS

Earlier in this chapter I explained that the two sources of infection with the AIDS virus are blood and sexual intercourse. By now, we have learned to prevent infections through blood by testing it before it is used. But the bigger of the two problems remains: short of chastity or 100 percent monogamy, can you be safe? Here is what can be done to minimize the possibility of infection.

Sexual relations with someone who has had sex with multiple or anonymous partners increases risk and, if this fact is known or suspected, the following precautions should be taken.

An exchange of body fluids should be avoided—particularly when having intimate relations with someone who might have used I.V. drugs in the past or who may have been a practicing homosexual or bisexual.

If initiating a new sexual relationship with someone whose past is unknown, sexual activities should be limited to those that do not permit an exchange of body secretions. During intercourse, condoms should be used—consistently. One has to keep in mind that even a single sexual experience with an AIDS-infected person is sufficient to transmit the virus.

Condoms do block the AIDS virus, which may be present in semen, vaginal secretions, or blood, and can be transmitted during vaginal, oral, or anal sex. Earlier, I mentioned that the use of a spermicidal jelly can improve the effectiveness of a condom used to prevent infection.

To use a condom properly, unroll it over the erect penis, leaving about half an inch of slack at the tip to hold the semen when it is ejaculated. The condom should be put on before the penis makes any contact with any of the woman's orifices. To reduce the possibility of tearing the condom, a water soluble lubricant (such as vaginal or surgical jelly) should be used. Oil-based lubricants like petroleum jelly should be avoided since they weaken latex. Should the condom leak or shrink, douching with lots of warm water may help to flush out virus-containing material.

Condoms are now sold in many varieties of colors and shapes. They come with ribbed or rough ridges; dry or prelub-ricated; and in a choice of plain tip or reservoir end. There are still other condoms that are made from animal membranes rather than latex—usually lamb gut. However, these are quite a bit more expensive and less reliable and should not be used for the prevention of AIDS. Condoms do not come in different sizes.

It is best to purchase condoms in a store whose merchandise is likely to turn over frequently, as these devices can lose some of their dependability with age. If possible, they should be stored in a cool place. This excludes the glove compartment of a car during warm months.

In male homosexual relationships, the passive recipient partner in anal intercourse is exposed to much greater risk, which can be reduced by use of a condom.

In long-term monogamous heterosexual relationships where there is no history of drug use, the risk of an infection is exceedingly small so there is no need to use condoms merely for the purpose of preventing such an infection, unless one of the partners suffers from recurring herpes or some other recurring, sexually transmissible infection.

If a "new" relationship survives an initial period of, say, five to six months, can a couple safely discontinue the use of condoms or other precautions? If not, when can they do so?

That is a question without a single answer. Every relationship is different. One would need to know how accurate each person's recollection is of his or her recent sexual history. And, is there any possibility of some dalliance outside the supposedly monogamous relationship? Ideally, a couple, after six months, should have serological tests. Practically speaking, however, if enough personal trust and mutual knowledge have been established for the risk to be minimal or unlikely, such testing may be unnecessary. But too many variables affect a relationship for there to be a definitive answer to the question of how soon precautions against AIDS may be abandoned.

Incidentally, such a thing as a "false positive" test result is virtually nonexistent when it comes to AIDS. It has happened—but so rarely that it should not enter into the individual's decision about having a blood test.

The Safety Of Blood Transfusions

Since donations are now rejected from persons with histories of having been in a high risk group at any time, transfused blood is almost totally safe. I say "almost" because there is something known as a "window period," a time span of, at most, six months after infection has taken place, when the blood may still test negative for viral antibodies—the indications looked for in a test that would indicate whether an infection has occurred.

Because of this minute factor, which makes it impossible to say that donated blood is 100 percent safe, blood banks are encouraging the donation and storage of one's own blood for transfusion when elective (non-urgent) surgery is planned and time permits. This is an excellent idea, although the cost of storing one's own blood in liquid state might be prohibitively high for some people. Long-term frozen storage, the alternative to liquid storage, is not generally recommended because such blood would not be readily available in an emergency.

If Your Blood Tests Positive For AIDS

Though this may seem small consolation at the traumatic moment when you learn that you have tested positive and are an AIDS reactor, you should know that there are between one and two million people in the U.S. and many millions more around the globe who share your misfortune. All over the world, research on treatment and a cure for AIDS has a top priority with scientists, governments, private health agencies, foundations, and universities. No one can foresee the future, but with so much research underway a breakthrough is bound to come.

Furthermore, though a reactor, you may never develop the disease AIDS. So try to maintain a positive attitude. Optimism is a big factor in an individual's fight against any illness.

Behavior Modification For Those Who Test Positive

It is just common sense and decency for people who are positive reactors to modify their sexual behavior in ways that will prevent them from transmitting the infection to others and prevent them from contracting yet another S.T.D., which could further impair the body's immune system.

If celibacy is out of the question, then frankness with a new partner is a must. Seemingly, however, sexual intercourse with another person who is also a reactor is not contraindicated, although the final answer on that score is not yet in. Only time will tell for sure whether complications can develop as a result of two reactors having sexual relations. In all cases, "protected" sex should be the rule, whether one or both partners are infected.

Women reactors should avoid pregnancy until answers are found on how to prevent infection of the embryo or newborn. It is also believed that pregnancy can escalate the progress of the disease more quickly than any other known factor—with pregnant women going rapidly from asymptomatic carriers to having the disease AIDS.

Getting AIDS Counseling

The response of an individual to test results is unpredictable. But every positive reactor, whether or not the disease develops, should have AIDS counseling and, in some cases, a complete medical evaluation. Every state has set up special counseling services with people specially trained to give advice on how to best cope with circumstances as they develop. In some instances, psychological counseling may be indicated if the individual is extremely anxious and depressed—which is not uncommon.

A Positive Reactor To AIDS Is No Threat To Friends, Families And Co-Workers

Since AIDS can be transmitted only through blood and sexual activities, a reactor cannot infect people at home, in the workplace, or in a social or public environment. If blood is not offered for donation (it would be rejected anyway) and there is no exchange of body fluids, no one's health is threatened by someone infected with the AIDS virus.

This virus does not spread through casual social or household contact. There is no danger of acquiring it from a co-worker who is a carrier. Bathrooms and toilet seats are safe. So is sharing everything from a glass to a house. Nor can AIDS be transmitted through touching, hugging, shaking hands, sweating, cooking, sneezing, or just being close friends. Also, there is no transmission within families or between people sharing a house, unless, of course, there are sexual relations.

Even people who have the actual disease AIDS and who are not just asymptomatic carriers of the virus are no threat to friends and co-workers since the symptoms they show are manifestations of other infections that need be of little concern to those with intact immune systems.

It would seem that the human skin is a good barrier against the virus. In hospitals, even those who have been accidentally stuck with infected needles very rarely develop positive blood tests or signs of AIDS infections.

As this book goes to press, we have knowledge of only two instances of para-professionals working with AIDS patients who have developed the disease. Reports on these instances indicate that there may have been an accidental exchange of body fluids (non-sexual) between the patient and the para-professional treating him.

Anti-Discrimination Laws

Unlike other communicable diseases, such as chicken pox or the flu, this infection is not transmitted through casual contact, as I have pointed out repeatedly. Hence, a number of states, thus far, have legally prohibited discrimination against AIDS patients. In addition to Washington, D.C., these states are California, Colorado, Connecticut, Florida, Illinois, Maine, Maryland, Massachusetts, Missouri, New Jersey, New Mexico, New York, Ohio, Oregon, Pennsylvania, Rhode Island, Washington, and West Virginia.

What People Know vs. What People Do

Despite widespread fear of the AIDS infection, there is a wide gap between what people know and what people do, as far as their sexual activities are concerned. While large-scale interviews show that people have reduced their number of sexual partners and that the use of condoms has increased, the occurrence of other reportable sexually transmitted diseases has not shown the expected decline. This may be due, in part, to the fact that some population segments are difficult to reach through education, particularly those who use injected drugs.

And Now For Some Encouraging Facts . . .

Although I have mentioned this before, it cannot be emphasized too often in this era of near-panic within some high risk groups: *of those infected with the virus, the majority may never develop the actual disease AIDS*. It is too early to know what percentage will remain permanently asymptomatic. For example, in one study that followed up infected males for six years, only 13 percent developed AIDS symptoms. In other studies, however, the percentages were higher. One study showed that 33 percent developed AIDS during a six-year period. For those who are diagnosed as AIDS positive but asymptomatic, six years is a long time, during which much progress may be made in suppressing the virus.

The other good news is that, among heterosexual couples—with the exception of I.V. drug users—the likelihood of getting AIDS, even from casual sexual encounters, is still exceedingly small. This fact should not deter couples from taking the precautionary measures described in this chapter since, unfortunately, the small chance of acquiring the AIDS disease is offset by the serious consequences should it happen.

CHAPTER NINETEEN

Getting Tests
And Treatment

If, despite all caution, you develop a sexually transmitted disease, by all means have it treated promptly, if treatment is possible. Not to do so can endanger your health and even your life. In the case of people who develop AIDS or who are symptomatic but react positively to the AIDS virus, counseling is also recommended.

If you have a personal physician, you can go to him or her with equanimity. Doctors today see people of all ages and backgrounds who are suffering from one or another of the S.T.D.s, and you can feel confident that you won't be looked upon with horror just because you have, or think you have, one of these diseases.

If you don't have a private physician, or choose not to go that route, you can go to a public health clinic. On the following pages you will find the telephone numbers of state health departments that you can call to get the address of the public clinic nearest you. Most of these clinics are either free or charge nominal fees, and since they specialize in S.T.D.s, you can expect to be treated by experienced, knowledgeable personnel.

Failure to seek treatment for an S.T.D. is sometimes based on denial, embarrassment, or the hope that the infection will go away on its own. S.T.D.s rarely do that. They should be diagnosed and, for most of these infections, the sooner treatment is initiated, the better. Prompt treatment will lessen the possibility of residual damage.

The S.T.D. division of each state health department can provide you with advice on where confidential testing for AIDS can be done. There is definitely a need for wider, voluntary testing (always with assurance of confidentiality) among those who believe they have good reason for concern. If you are among these people and see a doctor for any other reason, he or she—whether in a private office, a clinic, or a hospital—should be aware of your concern about AIDS and, if you've already been tested, the doctor should be told the result of such tests.

How To Locate An S.T.D. Treatment Center

Your local health department will usually be able to give you the address of the nearest public health clinic where you can be treated for an S.T.D. or tested for AIDS. If you live in a small town that doesn't have such a facility, call your state health department, tell them where you live, and ask for the address and clinic hours of the venereal disease clinic nearest you.

Here is a list of phone numbers for such state information centers:

● Alabama	205/261-5131	● Montana	406/444-4740
● Alaska	907/561-4233	● Nebraska	402/471-2937
● Arizona	602/255-1200	● Nevada	702/885-4988
● Arkansas	501/661-2395	● New Hampshire	603/271-4487
● California	916/445-0553	● New Jersey	609/588-3520
● Colorado	303/331-8320	● New Mexico	505/827-3201
● Connecticut	203/566-5058	● New York	518/473-0641
● Delaware	302/995-8422	● North Carolina	919/733-3419
● District of		● North Dakota	701/224-2378
Columbia	202/332-2437	● Ohio	614/466-4673
● Florida	904/488-2905	● Oklahoma	405/271-4061
● Georgia	800/342-2437	● Oregon	503/229-5792
● Hawaii	808/548-5986	● Pennsylvania	717/787-3350
● Idaho	208/334-5944	● Puerto Rico	809/721-4050
● Illinois	312/871-5696	● Rhode Island	401/277-2362
● Indiana	317/633-8406	● South	
● Iowa	515/281-5424	Carolina	803/758-5534
● Kansas	913/862-9360	● South Dakota	605/773-3364
● Kentucky	502/564-4478	● Tennessee	901/576-7714
● Louisiana	504/528-2437	● Texas	512/458-7328
● Maine	207/289-3747	● Utah	801/533-6191
● Maryland	301/945-2437	● Vermont	802/863-7240
● Massachusetts	617/522-3700	● Virginia	804/786-6267
● Michigan	517/373-1396	● Washington	206/361-2914
● Minnesota	612/623-5414	● West Virginia	304/348-5358
● Mississippi	205/261-5131	● Wisconsin	608/267-8739
● Missouri	816/353-9902	● Wyoming	307/777-7953

CHAPTER TWENTY

15 Questions Frequently Asked About Prevention and Treatment

There are certain questions about prevention and treatment of S.T.D.s that are frequently asked of clinicians—they come up over and over again. These are the 15 most frequently asked questions, along with the answers to them.

1. What Can I Do To Protect Myself Against S.T.D.s?

You might practice prudence and selectivity. Both help.

But putting these aside, I will tell you once again that the good ol' condom is quite effective—at least against gonorrhea, chlamydia, AIDS, and, to a lesser degree, herpes. I realize that condoms are not terribly popular among men, but they can protect you against lesions that are right on the parts most involved in the action.

In contrast to influenza, dysentery, and some other general infections, S.T.D.s *can* be prevented. Naturally, no one will get such a disease who shuns all sex contacts. This, of course, is not recommended for mature people. However, sexually active individuals can avoid an S.T.D. by being monoga- mous—having sexual relations with only one person known to be in good health.

Beyond that, it becomes a matter of reducing the *likelihood* of getting an infection. The risk can be reduced by practicing monogamy, at least *periodically*, and by being cautious in choosing a mate. Every reduction in the turnover rate will increase the odds against S.T.D.s. People who consider sex as an activity to be engaged in whenever the opportunity pre- sents itself, must recognize that every sport, whether it's ski- ing, football, or car racing, carries with it a certain rate of risk, and in this instance, a rather high one.

2. If I Do Have A Casual Sexual Experience, Is There Something I Can Do To Lessen The Likelihood Of An S.T.D.?

If you're looking for a protective device or technique that is entirely effective, there isn't one. If you think, however, that you may have been exposed to infection, there are a couple of things you might do. A man should empty his blad- der right after intercourse and immediately wash his penis and genital area with soap and water. A woman should also wash thoroughly and, if possible, use a low-pressure douche consist- ing of a quart of warm water and, if available, a tablespoon of ordinary vinegar. These things might help in prevention but none of them can be entirely relied upon—certainly not in the case of AIDS.

3. Are Prostitutes A Common Source of S.T.D.s?

Years ago, they were a prime source of infection. Nowadays, however, prostitution is experiencing a business slump except in some special situations, such as in large cities and around army posts, particularly overseas. The competition by non-professionals and para-professionals is keenly felt by the regular pros and estimates range that from only 5 percent to 10 percent of the new cases of S.T.D.s are being spread by prostitutes.

In countries where prostitutes are the principal source of sexually transmitted diseases, it seems easier to control them with frequent physical examinations. This does have its severe limitations, though, because an infection can be acquired the day after an examination. Furthermore, a disease may be communicable before a test will show a positive result.

4. Can You Develop Immunity To S.T.D.s?

There is no such immunity. Except, of course, somebody who is already infected with syphilis or AIDS cannot acquire a new, or primary infection while the old infection is still with him. But as soon as a person is cured of an S.T.D., he or she is physically able to acquire one or another infection again. Sometimes there may not be overt signs of such a reinfection, but the organisms, if present, are still capable of being transferred to someone else.

5. When I Go For A Gynecological Or Other Routine Medical Checkup, Does The Doctor Automatically Examine Me For An S.T.D.?

Not ordinarily. Even gynecologists don't routinely check for such diseases. However, if this is even remotely on your mind, you'd better mention it and don't be shy about it. Your doctor is faced with this consideration day-in, day-out. Of course, if any symptoms you describe, or any signs he or she can observe, point towards an S.T.D., then the doctor would very likely test for it. But often such symptoms are absent. During pregnancy, however, tests are routinely done for syphilis and often for gonorrhea, whether the patient asks for them or not.

6. What Is A Pap Test And What's Its Connection With S.T.D.s?

A Pap test is an examination to determine if there are cancer cells on the cervix; that is, the tip of the womb. This test was introduced by a physician by the name of Papanicolaou over thirty years ago. Since the test came into wide use it has cut down on the death rate from cancer of the cervix.

In doing the test, the doctor scrapes a little material from the tip of the womb where it protrudes into the vagina. He or she transfers this material to a glass slide and the rest of the work is done in a laboratory. There, a pathologist reads the slide and determines if there are cancer cells, suspicious cells of any kind, or anything else that might prove troublesome in the future.

But a Pap test is *not* a test for S.T.D.s, with two exceptions: where trichomonas may be found, or where there are indications of the presence of herpes on the cervix.

7. When You Get A Pap Test, Is It Automatically Accompanied By Tests For S.T.D.s?

A few physicians do this routinely, but don't count on it. Don't have the slightest reluctance, however, to tell your doctor that you'd like to have "a culture for gonorrhea," or tests for other infections, added to the examination. Your doctor probably won't bat an eye and it's the sensible thing for you to do if you have even the remotest cause for concern.

Nowadays, many clinics do automatically add such a test when women come in for other reasons. This is known as "screening." The screening procedure has, in the past, successfully contributed to the control of TB—people were automatically given chest x-rays when they came into clinics, hospitals, or some private medical offices, even though they had come in for reasons other than a chest infection. If everyone could be screened for gonorrhea, for example, we could control the epidemic. But it's unlikely that this will ever happen.

8. What Is Meant By A Premarital Examination For An S.T.D.?

Some states require a physical examination of both prospective bride and groom in order to prevent syphilis in the offspring. Since syphilis is one of the most crippling infections an embryo can acquire from its mother while nesting in the womb, this requirement is understandable. Most states require only a blood test for syphilis. Those states that also ask for a physical examination, do so to enable a doctor to look for syphilis signs of a very early sort, perhaps a chancre that might be present before the blood could show a positive reading. However, most physicians rely on the blood test alone. These premarital laws do not call for tests for other S.T.D.s. So, except where special indications suggest them, few physicians will include them as part of the premarital examination.

One out of every eighty-one applicants for a marriage license is found to have a positive reaction to the blood test for syphilis. This is a national figure which varies considerably in different parts of the country. The denser the population, the poorer the people, and, in general, the farther south one goes, the greater is the frequency of such tests revealing syphilis.

Occasionally, such tests are what we call "reactive," which means positive—despite the fact that there is no presence of, or past history of syphilis. These are known as "false positive" results and they don't at all mean that the laboratory has made a mistake or done a poor job. Such false positive results simply occur in a small percentage of tests. Under such circumstances, the clinician or doctor has to use good judgment and tact in explaining this to the patient, and in deciding whether to do further tests.

In the case of a couple already expecting a baby, it makes no sense to postpone the marriage until further tests, and possibly treatment, can be initiated. But even with a pregnant parent, these tests for syphilis have to be done—if infection does exist, steps can be taken, and treatment given, to protect the health of the unborn.

On a voluntary basis, an AIDS test can be requested. As yet, no state requires it.

9. How Long After Obtaining Evidence Of A Negative Blood Test Can That Test Be Used To Get A Marriage License?

In many states, a certificate showing the results of a blood test for syphilis cannot be more than forty days old in order for a marriage license to be issued. If you're planning to be married, telephone your local marriage license bureau or health department to find out the requirements in the state where you plan to wed.

10. Are There Any Immunizations Against S.T.D.s?

There are none in existence at this time. Despite ongoing research and experiments to develop such vaccines, the chances are not very good for their early availability. The reason for this is that there are no preventive inoculations against diseases that don't produce a lasting immunity. There are vaccines against measles, smallpox, typhoid, and many other infections—but each of these is a disease where you build up a permanent immunity after you have had the natural disease itself. Such is not the case with S.T.D.s. Even if some now-unforeseen development should make a vaccine available, the effectiveness would probably be short-lived.

Only with syphilis is the situation somewhat different. A vaccine might be developed but it would interfere with the results of syphilis blood tests. After someone was inoculated with the vaccine, we might not be able to tell if he or she actually had a case of syphilis or had developed a reactive (positive) blood test because of the inoculation.

The same can be said about AIDS. Both in the U.S. and elsewhere, the search is intense to develop a vaccine. But who will want to take it? One inherent negative of such a vaccine, should it be developed, is that one's blood test may become positive and one wouldn't know if it were due to the vaccine or to an infection.

One exception in this bleak outlook is the development of a vaccine against hepatitis B. This is described in the chapter on S.T.D.s among homosexuals (Chapter 17). The reason for this isolated exception is that an attack of hepatitis B confers lifelong immunity.

11. Why Is It Necessary For A Doctor To Report Certain Cases Of V.D. To The Public Health Authorities?

Let's take syphilis first. This is so important a disease and can be of such serious consequences for those infected with it, that public health authorities try to track each case to its source. This is done, however, with the knowledge and cooperation of the person who first came in to be treated. It cannot be done without his or her cooperation. When contacts or "sources" are found, they are encouraged to have treatment in the interest of their own health and that of others with whom they will have contact. Then, the contacts of *those* people are sought out for treatment, and so on down the line.

With gonorrhea and the other S.T.D.s you have a different story. There is little tracing of sources because it's so difficult to do. The disease spreads too fast, there are too many of them, and few public health agencies would have staffs large enough to undertake the job of following up all sources. Just the same, it's necessary for private physicians to report cases of gonorrhea to public health authorities so that they will know how widespread this communicable disease is in any one area, what general measures need to be taken to cope with it, and when to follow up, selectively, if indicated.

As with any communicable disease, educational steps and budgeting considerations are influenced, if not actually determined, by reports on the prevalence of the disease. If the various funding agencies didn't know how much S.T.D. was around, they would surely cut out the funding for the clinics that treat patients with such illnesses.

The situation with AIDS is different. Unfortunately, there is still a stigma attached to this disease, so a patient's desire for anonymity is respected.

12. Are There Any State Where Doctors Are *Not* Required To Report Certain S.T.D.s?

The laws in all fifty states require that gonorrhea and syphilis cases be reported. Of course, each patient has an assurance of confidentiality. If contacts are traced in syphilis cases, it's done with the knowledge and cooperation of the person who first came in for treatment.

In this country, the other S.T.D.s are not reportable. However, in some European countries, non-gonococcal urethritis and herpes have to be reported to the health authorities.

Certain infections that may or may not be acquired through sexual contact—including amebiasis, shigella, and salmonella—have to be reported in the U.S.

13. If, Despite All Caution, I Do Get An S.T.D., What Should I Do?

Get treatment, of course.

Apart from that, you should let your sexual contact know that you have become infected so that he or she can also seek treatment. Even if you never want to have anything to do with that person again, you should be decent enough to inform him or her. Also, and this is very important: avoid any sexual contact until your physician says that your infection is not in a communicable stage.

Of course, generally speaking, from here on your threshold of suspicion should be lowered. In other words, you should become more cautious about whom you select for sexual involvement. Common sense would tell you to increase the degree to which you assess, and possibly reject, opportunities for sexual relations.

14. Where Is The Best Place To Go For Treatment?

You have a choice. Whether you are sure you have an S.T.D. or not, you can go for a consultation to your family doctor, to an internist, to a gynecologist, to a urologist, or to a specialist in infectious diseases. In addition, most cities have free health department clinics. You can find out where such clinics are located by calling your local or state health department.

In this country, few private practitioners make a specialty of treating S.T.D.s, although there are specialists in "infectious diseases." Health department clinics, on the other hand, usually offer treatment without charge—and their staffs have a great deal of specialized experience with these diseases. In Europe, dermatologists include S.T.D.s in their specialties. In the U.S. and Canada, this applies only to a limited number of skin specialists.

15. Do Minors Need Parental Consent To Be Treated For S.T.D.s?

A minor does not need parental consent to be examined and treated for S.T.D.s. This is now true in all fifty states. Furthermore, parents will not be notified of such examination or treatment.

A Glossary of Terms

Amebiasis. A disease caused by amoeba (ameba). Usually affects the intestinal tract, but amoeba may invade other organ systems as well.

Amoeba. An intestinal parasite, a one-celled micro-organism, usually acquired through food or drink. However, it is also sexually transmissible.

Antibody. A substance that the body develops to fight an invading micro-organism.

Arthritis. An inflammation of joints.

Asymptomatic. Having a disease without showing signs of it.

Bacteria. Microscopic organisms classified as plants. They are able to live in the soil, in animals, in man, and practically anywhere in organic nature. Bacteria appear in many shapes: round, rod-like, spiral, and others.

Candida. A yeast-like fungus, frequently found in the vagina. Its presence may produce symptoms of greatly varying intensity.

Canker sores. Ulcerations on the mucous lining of the mouth or lips, sometimes confused with herpes sores. These are not caused by the herpes virus.

Carcinoma. Cancer.

Carriers. In connection with communicable diseases, refers to infected individuals who can transmit a disease but who have no symptoms or evidence of the disease-producing agent they carry.

CDC. Centers for Disease Control, located in Atlanta, Georgia. The national government agency that, among other functions, tracks epidemics and assists in solving problems presented by obscure outbreaks of illnesses.

Cervicitis. An inflammation of the tip of the womb.

Cervix. The tip of the womb; protrudes into the vagina.

Chancre. An ulcer, usually painless, of fairly hard, rubbery consistency, and the first apparent manifestation of syphilis.

Chancroid. A sexually transmitted disease characterized by a painful ulceration and caused by the Ducrey bacillus.

Chlamydia. A minute, living organism that shares some characteristics with viruses, others with bacteria. Produces an S.T.D. similar to gonorrhea.

Coliform. Coliform bacteria, commonly found in the intestines. They may be disease-producing if they invade other organ systems such as the bladder or the Fallopian tubes.

Condyloma. Another term for warts. Broadly based condyloma are usually due to syphilis and are then termed condyloma lata. The non-syphilitic type is called condyloma acuminata (sharp-pointed).

Congenital syphilis. Syphilis acquired by the fetus while in the womb.

Conjunctivae. The red mucuous membrane which lines the eyelids and part of the eyeball.

Conjunctivitis. An inflammation of the conjunctivae, usually due to an infection.

Cortisone. A hormone produced by the shell of the adrenal gland.

Cryptitis. A term usually applied to an inflammation of the small recesses and grooves within the rectal and anal walls.

Culture. The growth of micro-organisms in artificial media. A specimen is put on a medium that supports the growth of bacteria, if any are present, and placed in the atmosphere of an incubator.

Cyst. An enclosed space, within a membrane, filled with liquid or semi-solid material.

Cystitis. An inflammation of the bladder.

Cytomegalovirus. A common virus, related to the herpes family of viruses, that may or may not produce disease in humans, depending on individual susceptibility.

Darkfield examination. A system using a special condenser that transmits only light entering its periphery, so that certain particles are illuminated and glow against a dark background. It is used to determine the presence of the spirochaete which causes syphilis.

Discharge. In reference to sexually transmitted diseases, the emission of a substance from the vagina or penis in quantities beyond the normal range.

Ectopic pregnancy. Implantation of a fertilized egg in a Fallopian tube instead of in the uterus.

Endocarditis. Inflammation of the inner lining of the heart.

Epidemic. An outbreak usually involving the rapid spread of an infectious disease.

Epidemiology. The science or knowledge of the prevalence and transmission of diseases of public health significance.

Epididymitis. An inflammation of the organ that hugs the testicles.

Epstein-Barr virus. A virus within the herpes family of viruses that causes infectious mononucleosis.

Facultative pathogens. Organisms that are capable of coexisting with other organisms in the vagina but that can produce disease, given circumstances favorable to them.

Fallopian tubes. The channels that link the ovaries with the womb, and through which an egg is transported to the uterus where it will normally nest, if fertilized. Serious consequences result when the egg is implanted in the tube.

False positive. When applied to syphilis tests, it means that the test is reactive, as if a syphilitic infection were present, when, in fact, the "positivity" is due to some other cause.

Fellatio. Sexual stimulation of the penis by oral contact.

Fertility. The ability to reproduce.

Fissure. A lineal fault; in other words, a crack in the skin or a mucous membrane.

Fistula. An abnormal canal that may form as the result of an abscess or from a chronic infection.

Folliculitis. An inflammation or infection of hair follicles.

Gamma globulin. An older term for Immunoglobulin—a protein produced by the body, essential in the defense against infections. Used clinically in the form of injections to prevent some infections.

Gardnerella vaginalis. A micro-organism frequently found in the vagina. May cause an inflammation of the vagina although it often produces no symptoms. Formerly known as haemophilus vaginalis.

Genital warts. *See condyloma.*

Giardia. A one-celled micro-organism that can cause a chronic illness localized in the intestines. Usually transmitted through drinking water but also sexually transmitted.

Gonococcus. The micro-organism causing gonorrhea.

Gonorrhea. A common, infectious, sexually transmitted disease caused by the gonococcus.

Gram stain. A laboratory procedure that facilitates the distinction of bacteria. Depending on their staining characteristics, bacteria are designated Gram-positive or Gram-negative organisms.

Granuloma inguinale. A chronic, sexually transmitted disease, characterized by swelling and ulcerations and the presence in microscopic examination of "Donovan bodies."

Hepatitis. Inflammation of the liver.

Herpes. Name of a group of infections. The term originally referred to diseases characterized by the appearance of small blisters, a manifestation that may be missing in some infections of the herpes group.

Herpes progenitalis. Herpes around the genital area.

Herpes simplex. A viral disease characterized by an eruption of minute blisters on a red base. This disease tends to recur in the same area of the body.

Herpes zoster (Shingles). Painful skin eruption along the lines of a nerve trunk. Caused by the same virus that produces chicken pox in children.

Immunity. Resistance against an infection.

Incubation period. The time period from the moment when an infection is acquired to the appearance of the first symptom.

Infectious mono. *See mononucleosis.*

Intra-uterine device. A contraceptive device placed within the uterine cavity to prevent the embedding of a fertilized egg.

Jaundice. Abnormal yellowness of the skin or mucous membranes due to excessive amounts of bilirubin (bile pigment) in the blood.

Kaposi's sarcoma. A disease related to cancer and characterized by multiple bluish-purple tumors or nodules, and a tendency to internal bleeding. Diagnosis is made or confirmed with the aid of microscope slides.

Labia. The larger outer lip and the smaller inner lip at the entrance of the vagina.

Lesion. The visible sign of a skin disease.

Lues. Another name for syphilis.

Luetic. One who has Lues, or syphilis.

Lymph nodes. Small, round, or oval nodes scattered throughout the body. Contain cells that play a major role in defending the body against infections.

Lymphogranuloma venereum. A chronic, sexually transmitted, infectious disease caused by a micro-organism of the chlamydia group. Commonly abbreviated as LGV.

Malaise. A generally uncomfortable feeling of impaired health, usually without reference to a specific organ of the body.

Meatitis. An inflammation of the male urethra at the tip of the penis.

Meatus. With reference to S.T.D.s, usually refers to the tip of the penis.

Micro-organism. An organism or live substance too small to be seen without magnification.

Mite. A minute animal with eight legs, related to the spider family. Some species of mites produce disease in humans and animals.

Monilia. A yeast-like organism, the same as candida, frequently inhabiting the vagina and occasionally causing a disease named Moniliasis.

Moniliasis. An inflammation or disease caused by the micro-organism monilia. In the fungus family.

Mononucleosis. An infectious disease caused by the Epstein-Barr virus. Involves the blood or tissues.

Mycoplasma. A type of minute micro-organism without cell walls. Can cause disease in humans and animals but is also capable of living within the organism without causing disease.

Neisseria gonorrhea. The scientific name of the bacterium that causes gonorrhea.

Neuro-syphilis. Syphilitic infection of the nervous system. Symptoms usually appear many years after the original infection.

Non-gonococcal urethritis. An infection of the male urethra caused by organisms other than the gonococcus. It includes chlamydial urethritis and urethritis due to other, often undetermined micro-organisms.

Non-gonococcal urethritis. An infection of the male urethra caused by organisms other than the gonococcus. It includes chlamydial urethritis and urethritis due to other, often undetermined micro-organisms.

Non-specific vaginitis. An inflammation or irritation of the vagina (usually accompanied by symptoms such as itching or discharge) where no specific causative agent can be isolated or identified.

P.I.D. Abbreviation for Pelvic Inflammatory Disease.

Pap test. Microscopic examination of a scraping from the cervix, primarily serving as an early diagnostic procedure of cervical cancer.

Pediculosis. Infection with lice.

Pelvic inflammatory disease. An infection of the Fallopian tubes, often involving additional, adjoining organs such as the ovaries or the inner lining of the abdomen (peritoneum).

Penicillin. The first antibiotic produced from a mold. Highly effective against syphilis and the gonococcus.

Peri-hepatitis. An inflammation of the membranes that surround the liver. An occasional complication of gonorrhea and chlamydial infections.

Peritoneoscope. An optical instrument introduced through the skin into the abdominal cavity, for diagnostic or surgical purposes.

Peritoneum. The lining of the organs in the abdomen.

Peritonitis. An inflammation of the lining of the abdominal organs.

pH. Technically speaking, this refers to the hydrogen concentration of a substance. Practically, it indicates the degree of acidity or alkalinity. A pH above 7 represents alkalinity; below 7, acidity. The lower the pH, the greater the acidity. The scale runs from zero to 14, with 7 representing neutrality.

Placebo. A substance given as medication but which is known to have neither beneficial nor adverse effects.

Pneumocystis Carinii. Related to AIDS, a kind of pneumonia caused by a parasitic infection in the lungs.

Proctitis. An inflammation of the anal canal.

Prodrome. The earliest symptoms, preceding the outbreak of an illness.

Prostate. A gland located below the male bladder and producing much of the fluid in which the sperm cells are suspended.

Prostatitis. An inflammation of the prostate gland.

Psittacosis. An infection similar to pneumonia, found in birds and rarely transmitted to humans. Caused by a micro-organism of the chlamydia group. When acquired by humans, it is usually from such birds as parrots, parakeets, ducks, pigeons, and turkeys.

Pubic lice. A species of lice that infests the pubic hair predominantly and is, thereby, readily transmissible during sexual intercourse.

Reactive. Showing a positive reaction to a test. In particular, suggestive of syphilis.

Reactor. A person having a positive reaction to a test; as, for instance, to a syphilis or AIDS test.

Reiter's syndrome. An illness with symptoms of urethritis, conjunctivitis and arthritis.

Remission. The subsiding of symptoms in diseases that tend to recur.

Reportable diseases. A limited list of illnesses of public health significance that must be reported by physicians and clinicians to health authorities. Syphilis and gonorrhea are reportable diseases; herpes is not.

Retrovir. Drug used to interfere with the virus, HIV, which causes AIDS. While this drug is administered on a selective basis, it has not been approved for all manifestations of AIDS, and is not considered a cure.

S.T.D. Sexually Transmitted Disease. An infection acquired through the close contact of cohabitation or sexual contact.

Salmonella. A micro-organism that commonly causes internal infections. May also be found in other organs of the body and can be sexually transmitted.

Salpingitis. An inflammation of one or both Fallopian tubes.

Scabies. An extremely itchy infection with mites that burrow canals in the skin.

Screening. Testing large groups of people for a specific disease for which they have shown no symptoms.

Serological test. A test done on the blood liquid, after removal of the cells suspended in it.

Serum hepatitis. An older term for what is now called hepatitis B.

Shedding. With reference to S.T.D.s, this term is used to describe the presence of viruses on the body surface, particularly from the site of a past or developing ulcer, even though there may be no visible manifestation of the ulcer itself.

Shigella. Bacteria that usually produce an acute illness of the lower intestine. Can be sexually transmitted.

Silent Reservoir. Carriers of infectious agents who are unaware of their infections.

Smear test. Small amount of discharge put on a slide, dried, stained and examined under the microscope.

Spirochaete. A coil-shaped micro-organism that causes syphilis and some other infectious diseases.

Sterility. In the context of sexually transmitted diseases, the inability to produce offspring due to organic changes produced by an infection.

Streptococcus. A common micro-organism with many subspecies. Some of these are harmless while others can produce serious infections in the throat or other organs of the body.

Stricture. Narrowing of an organ; in particular, a narrowing of the urethra or the anal canal.

Syphilis. An infectious disease caused by a corkscrew-shaped micro-organism.

Test of cure. A given treatment may or may not produce the destruction of the invading micro-organisms, and the disappearance of symptoms is not always evidence of cure. Lab tests carried out to ascertain whether the cure was successful are known as Tests of Cure.

Thrush. A whitish lining found on the surface of the mucous membranes and caused by the yeast-like fungus monilia.

Trachoma. An eye infection common in developing countries, particularly those with low sanitary standards. Caused by the same organism that produces chlamydia, the sexually transmitted disease.

Trichomonas. A micro-organism that is propelled by whip-like motion and can be readily observed under the microscope without staining the specimen.

Trichomoniasis. An infection with trichomonas.

Tumor. An abnormal growth of tissue.

Ulcer. A round or oval break in the skin or in a mucous membrane, due to a disease rather than to trauma.

Urethra. The exit duct from the bladder. In the male, serves as a duct through which sperm is emitted, as well as a carrier of urine from the bladder.

Urethritis. An inflammation usually due to an infection of the urethra.

Vaginitis. An irritation or inflammation of the vagina.

Venereal warts. Sexually transmitted warts that are usually somewhat softer and redder than the common warts seen on fingers.

Venus. In Roman mythology, the goddess of love and beauty.

Virus. A minute structure, much smaller than bacteria, that multiplies only within living cells. It causes illness in humans, animals, and plants.

Wassermann test. A test using blood serum to determine whether a person has or has had syphilis. The term "Wassermann," named after the man who first devised the test, is still used even though the original procedure has been modified.

Index

serology test, 87, 99, 144

shedding, 27, 30

shigella, 138, 191 *(also see Chapter 17.)*

shingles, *(see* herpes zoster*)*

silent reservoir, *(see* carriers*)*

silver nitrate, 107

skin, 68, 83, 95, 102, 117, 122 *(also see Chapter 15.)*

smear test, 19, 40, 68, 71, 140

socio-economic factors, 18, 46

Spectinomycin, 74

sperm, 98, 102, 106, 111, 141

sperm ducts, 17

spirochaete, 79, 85, 94

spleen, 101

sterility, 39, 67 *(also see* fertility*)*

streptococcus, 98, 109 *(also see Chapter 10.)*

stress, 24, 154

sulfa drugs, 73

sweating, 150

syphilis, 11, 14, 16, 19, 25, 26, 105, 107, 108, 115, 116, 125, 138, 145, 187, 188, 190 *(also see Chapter 8.)*

Tattoos, 18

test of cure, 73

testicles, 39, 67

tetracyclines, 40, 48, 53, 62, 74, 94, 96, 100, 109

throat, 27, 71, 83, 84, 101

thrush, 52, 53

Toxoplasma, 151

trachoma, 44

transfusions, 142, 159, 160, 161, 163, 174

travel, 19

treatment, 21, 41, 46, 48, 54, 55, 62, 73, 74, 75, 82, 88, 89, 94, 100, 109, 121, 129, 144, 155 *(also see Chapter 19.)*

trichomonas, trichomoniasis, 38, 52, 54, 97

tubes (Fallopian), 14, 17, 45, 59, 63, 70

Urethra, 37, 67, 70, 118, 121

urethritis, 13, 55 *(also see Chapter 3.)*

urination, 19, 45, 60, 66, 118, 119, 121

uterus, 45 *(also see* womb*)*

V.D., 11

VDRL test, 87

vaccines, 48, 99, 103, 143, 157

vagina, 27, 39, 51, 53, 56, 82, 95, 105, 112, 114, 118, 120

vaginitis, 94 *(also see Chapter 5.)*

venereal warts, 97, 125, 138, 145 *(also see Chapter 15.)*

Venus, 12

virus, 20, 24, 25, 38, 141

vomiting, 60

Wassermann test, 87

Western Blot Assay Test, 153

womb, 14, 60, 70, 72, 86, 108 *(also see* uterus)

Yaws, 91

youth, 18